Paramedic Care
Principles & Practice
Introduction to Paramedicine

Workbook

Fourth Edition

Paramedic Care
Principles & Practice
Introduction to Paramedicine

Workbook

Fourth Edition

ROBERT S. PORTER

REVISED BY

KEVIN T. COLLOPY, BA, FP-C, CCEMT-P, NREMT-P, WEMT

Performance Improvement & Education Coordinator
AirLink, VitaLink, & PCTS Specialty Care Transport
Lead Instructor, Wilderness Medical Associates
Wilmington, North Carolina

BRYAN E. BLEDSOE, DO, FACEP, FAAEM, EMT-P

Professor of Emergency Medicine
Director, Prehospital and Disaster Medicine Fellowship
University of Nevada School of Medicine
Attending Emergency Physician
University Medical Center of Southern Nevada
Medical Director, MedicWest Ambulance
Las Vegas, Nevada

ROBERT S. PORTER, MA, EMT-P

Senior Advanced Life Support Educator
Madison County Emergency Medical Services
Canastota, New York

RICHARD A. CHERRY, MS, NREMT-P

Director of Training
Northern Onondaga Volunteer Ambulance
Liverpool, New York

PEARSON

Boston Columbus Indianapolis New York San Francisco Upper Saddle River
Amsterdam Cape Town Dubai London Madrid Milan Munich Paris Montréal Toronto
Delhi Mexico City São Paulo Sydney Hong Kong Seoul Singapore Taipei Tokyo

Publisher: *Julie Levin Alexander*
Publisher's Assistant: *Regina Bruno*
Editor-in-Chief: *Marlene McHugh Pratt*
Senior Managing Editor for Development: *Lois Berlowitz*
Editorial Project Manager: *Triple SSS Press Media Development, Inc.*
Assistant Editor: *Jonathan Cheung*
Director of Marketing: *David Gesell*
Marketing Manager: *Brian Hoehl*
Marketing Specialist: *Michael Sirinides*
Managing Editor for Production: *Patrick Walsh*
Production Liaison: *Faye Gemmellaro*
Production Editor: *Muralidharan Krishnamurthy/S4Carlisle Publishing Services*
Manufacturing Manager: *Ilene Sanford*
Cover Design: *Kathryn Foot*
Cover Image: *© corepics/Shutterstock*
Composition: *S4Carlisle Publishing Services*
Cover and Interior Printer/Binder: *Edwards Brothers Malloy*

NOTICE ON CARE PROCEDURES

It is the intent of the authors and publisher that this Workbook be used as part of a formal Paramedic program taught by qualified instructors and supervised by a licensed physician. The procedures described in this Workbook are based upon consultation with EMT and medical authorities. The authors and publisher have taken care to make certain that these procedures reflect currently accepted clinical practice; however, they cannot be considered absolute recommendations.

The material in this Workbook contains the most current information available at the time of publication. However, federal, state, and local guidelines concerning clinical practices, including, without limitation, those governing infection control and universal precautions, change rapidly. The reader should note, therefore, that the new regulations may require changes in some procedures.

It is the responsibility of the reader to familiarize himself or herself with the policies and procedures set by federal, state, and local agencies as well as the institution or agency where the reader is employed. The authors and the publisher of this Workbook disclaim any liability, loss, or risk resulting directly or indirectly from the suggested procedures and theory, from any undetected errors, or from the reader's misunderstanding of the text. It is the reader's responsibility to stay informed of any new changes or recommendations made by any federal, state, or local agency as well as by his or her employing institution or agency.

NOTICE ON CPR AND ECC

The national standards for cardiopulmonary resuscitation (CPR) and emergency cardiovascular care (ECC) are reviewed and revised on a regular basis and may change slightly after this manual is printed. It is important that you know the most current procedures for CPR and ECC, both for the classroom and your patients. The most current information may be obtained from the appropriate credentialing agency.

Brady
is an imprint of

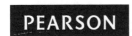

www.bradybooks.com

10 9 8 7 6 5 4 3 2 1
ISBN 10:   0-13-211232-9
ISBN 13:   978-0-13-211232-1

Dedication

This workbook is dedicated to the important people in your life: your wife/husband, mother, father, sister, brother . . . and friends who support you and the time and passion you devote to Emergency Medical Service.
Without them, this endeavor would be lonely and much less rewarding.

–ROBERT S. PORTER

Contents

INTRODUCTION

Welcome to the self-instructional Workbook for *Paramedic Care: Principles & Practice*. This Workbook is designed to help guide you through an educational program for initial or refresher training that follows the guidelines of the 2009 *National EMS Education Standards*. The Workbook is designed to be used either in conjunction with your instructor or as a self-study guide you use on your own.

This Workbook features many different ways to help you learn the material necessary to become a paramedic, as described next.

Features

Review of Chapter Objectives
Each chapter of *Paramedic Care: Principles & Practice* begins with objectives that identify the important information and principles addressed in the chapter reading. To help you identify and learn this material, each Workbook chapter reviews the important content elements addressed by these objectives as presented in the text.

Case Study Review
Each chapter of *Paramedic Care: Principles & Practice* includes a case study, introducing and highlighting important principles presented in the chapter. The Workbook reviews these case studies and points out much of the essential information and many of the applied principles they describe.

Content Self-Evaluation
Each chapter of *Paramedic Care: Principles & Practice* presents an extensive narrative explanation of the principles of paramedic practice. The Workbook chapter (or chapter section) contains between 10 and 50 multiple-choice questions to test your reading comprehension of the textbook material and to give you experience taking typical emergency medical service examinations.

Special Projects
The Workbook contains several projects that are special learning experiences designed to help you remember the information and principles necessary to perform as a paramedic. Special projects include crossword puzzles, fill-in-the-blank exercises, and a variety of other activities.

Content Review
The Workbook provides a comprehensive review of the material presented in Volume 1 of *Paramedic Care: Principles & Practice*. After the last text chapter has been covered, the Workbook presents an extensive content self-evaluation component that helps you recall and build upon the knowledge you have gained by reading the text, attending class, and completing the earlier Workbook chapters.

HOW TO USE THIS SELF-INSTRUCTIONAL WORKBOOK

The self-instructional Workbook accompanying *Paramedic Care: Principles & Practice* may be used as directed by your instructor or independently by you during your course of instruction. The following recommendations are intended to guide you in using the Workbook independently.

- Examine your course schedule and identify the appropriate text chapter or other assigned reading.

- Read the assigned chapter in *Paramedic Care: Principles & Practice* carefully. Do this in a relaxed environment, free of distractions, and give yourself adequate time to read and digest the material. The information presented in *Paramedic Care: Principles & Practice* is often technically complex and demanding, but it is very important that you comprehend it. Be sure that you read the chapter carefully enough to understand and remember what you have read.

- Carefully read the Review of Chapter Objectives at the beginning of each Workbook chapter (or section). This material includes both the objectives listed in *Paramedic Care: Principles & Practice* and narrative descriptions of their content. If you do not understand or remember what is discussed from your reading, refer to the referenced pages and reread them carefully. If you still do not feel comfortable with your understanding of any objective, consider asking your instructor about it.

- Reread the case study in *Paramedic Care: Principles & Practice*, and then read the Case Study Review in the Workbook. Note the important points regarding assessment and care that the Case Study Review highlights and be sure that you understand and agree with the analysis of the call. If you have any questions or concerns, ask your instructor to clarify the information.

- Take the Content Self-Evaluation at the end of each Workbook chapter (or section), answering each question carefully. Do this in a quiet environment, free from distractions, and allow yourself adequate time to complete the exercise. Correct your self-evaluation by consulting the answers at the back of the Workbook, and determine the percentage you have answered correctly (the number you got right divided by the total number of questions). If you have answered most of the questions correctly (85 to 90 percent), review those that you missed by rereading the material on the pages listed in the answer key and be sure you understand which answer is correct and why. If you have more than a few questions wrong (less than 85 percent correct), look for incorrect answers that are grouped together. This suggests that you did not understand a particular topic in the reading. Reread the text dealing with that topic carefully, and then retest yourself on the questions you got wrong. If incorrect answers are spread throughout the chapter content, reread the chapter and retake the Content Self-Evaluation to ensure that you understand the material. If you don't understand why your answer to a question is incorrect after reviewing the text, consult with your instructor.

- In a similar fashion, complete the exercises in the Special Projects section of the Workbook chapters (or sections). These exercises are specifically designed to help you learn and remember the essential principles and information presented in *Paramedic Care: Principles & Practice*.

- When you have completed this volume of *Paramedic Care: Principles & Practice* and its accompanying Workbook, prepare for a course test by reviewing both the text in its entirety and your class notes. Then take the Content Review examination in the Workbook. Again, review your score and any questions you have answered incorrectly by referring to the text and rereading the page or pages where the material is presented. If you note groupings of wrong answers, review the entire range of pages or the full chapter they represent.

    If, during your completion of the Workbook exercises, you have any questions that either the textbook or Workbook doesn't answer, write them down and ask your instructor about them. Prehospital emergency medicine is a complex and complicated subject, and answers are not always black and white. It is also common for different EMS systems to use differing methods of care. The questions you bring up in class, and your instructor's answers to them, will help you expand and complete your knowledge of prehospital emergency medical care.

GUIDELINES TO BETTER TEST-TAKING

The knowledge you will gain from reading the textbook, completing the exercises in the Workbook, listening in your paramedic class, and participating in your clinical and field experience will prepare you to care for patients who are seriously ill or injured. However, before you can practice these skills, you will have to pass several classroom written exams and your state's certification exam. Your performance on these exams will depend not only on your knowledge but also on your ability to answer test questions correctly. The following guidelines are designed to help your performance on tests and to better demonstrate your knowledge of pre-hospital emergency care.

1. Relax and be calm during the test.

A test is designed to measure what you have learned and to tell you and your instructor how well you are doing. An exam is not designed to intimidate or punish you. Consider it a challenge, and just try to do your best. Get plenty of sleep before the examination. Avoid coffee or other stimulants for a few hours before the exam, and be prepared.

Reread the text chapters, review the objectives in the Workbook, and review your class notes. It might be helpful to work with one or two other students and ask each other questions. This type of practice helps everyone better understand the knowledge presented in your course of study.

2. Read the questions carefully.

Read each word of the question and all the answers slowly. Words such as "except" or "not" may change the entire meaning of the question. If you miss such words, you may answer the question incorrectly even though you know the right answer.

Example:
The art and science of emergency medical services involves all of the following EXCEPT

    A. sincerity and compassion.
    B. respect for human dignity.
    C. placing patient care before personal safety.
    D. delivery of sophisticated emergency medical care.
    E. none of the above.

The correct answer is C, unless you miss the "EXCEPT."

3. Read each answer carefully.

Read each and every answer carefully. Although the first answer may be absolutely correct, so may the rest, and thus the best answer might be "all of the above."

Example:
Indirect medical direction is considered to be

    A. treatment protocols.
    B. training and education.
    C. quality assurance.
    D. chart review.
    E. all of the above.

Although answers A, B, C, and D are each correct, the best and only acceptable answer is "all of the above," E.

4. Delay answering questions you don't understand and look for clues.

When a question seems confusing or you don't know the answer, note it on your answer sheet and come back to it later. This will ensure that you have time to complete the test. You will also find that other questions on the test may give you hints to answer the one you've skipped over. It will also prevent you from being frustrated with an early question and letting it affect your performance.

Example:

Upon successful completion of a course of training as an EMT-P, most states will

 A. certify you. (correct)

 B. license you.

 C. register you.

 D. recognize you as a paramedic.

 E. issue you a permit.

Another question, later in the exam, may suggest the right answer:

The action of one state in recognizing the certification of another is called

 A. reciprocity. (correct)

 B. national registration.

 C. licensure.

 D. registration.

 E. extended practice.

5. Answer all questions.

Even if you do not know the right answer, do not leave a question blank. A blank question is always wrong, whereas a guess might be correct. If you can eliminate some of the answers as wrong, do so. It will increase the chances of a correct guess.

A multiple-choice question with five answers gives a 20 percent chance of a correct guess. If you can eliminate one or more incorrect answers, you increase your odds of a correct guess to 25 percent, 33 percent, and so on. An unanswered question has a 0 percent chance of being correct.

Just before turning in your answer sheet, check to be sure that you have not left any items blank.

Example:

When a paramedic is called by the patient (through the dispatcher) to the scene of a medical emergency, the medical direction physician has established a physician/patient relationship.

 A. True

 B. False

A true/false question gives you a 50 percent chance of a correct guess.

The hospital health professional(s) responsible for sorting patients as they arrive at the emergency department is/are usually the

 A. emergency physician.

 B. ward clerk.

 C. emergency nurse.

 D. trauma surgeon.

 E. both A and C (correct)

Paramedic Care
Principles & Practice
Introduction to Paramedicine

Workbook
Fourth Edition

Introduction to Paramedicine

Review of Chapter Objectives

With each chapter of the Workbook, we identify the objectives and the important elements of the textbook content. You should review these items and refer to the pages listed if any points are not clear.

After reading this chapter, you should be able to:

1. **Define key terms introduced in this chapter.**

   Knowing and being able to apply the key terms in each chapter is critical to understanding chapter concepts. Write the list of key terms. Then write the definition of each one in your own words. Check your understanding by confirming the definitions in the text glossary. Correct any misunderstandings. Create a study aid by writing each key term on the front of an index card and the definition on the back. Use the cards to quiz yourself or to have someone quiz you.

2. **Compare and contrast the roles of Emergency Medical Responders (EMRs), Emergency Medical Technicians (EMTs), and Advanced Emergency Medical Technicians (AEMTs) with the role of Paramedics in the emergency medical services system.** p. 3

   There are four recognized steps in the medical training of prehospital providers. These titles and their education are not unique to one another; rather each step up the training ladder builds on the foundation of the training before it. Similarly, the role of each provider is intimately linked to the others. Emergency Medical Responders (EMRs) represent those with the basic foundation of prehospital providers and are responsible for basic lifesaving skills until more advanced providers are available. The role of the EMR cannot be understated, though, because the EMR helps improve the lives of countless individuals who would become more gravely ill or injured, or even die, if EMRs were not available. The EMR works hand in hand with and learns from all other prehospital providers.

   Those wishing to take on additional training and responsibilities can become Emergency Medical Technicians (EMTs) whose education builds on the foundation set in EMR courses. The EMT learns additional basic life-supporting skills and gains a deeper understanding of the skills and information taught to the EMR. Traditionally, the EMT is the minimum training required to transport patients on an ambulance.

   Advanced Emergency Medical Technicians (AEMTs) are responsible for learning not only an in-depth understanding of all basic life-support skills, but they are also taught a limited number of advanced life-support skills that can be provided in the absence of, or under the supervision of, paramedics. The AEMT works closely with the other prehospital providers and must continue the interventions provided by the EMR and the EMT. AEMTs must understand why skills are performed in order to effectively provide their advanced interventions.

Paramedics are responsible for all aspects of patient care in the prehospital setting; however, their knowledge and capabilities are often greatly hampered unless they work closely with the EMR, EMT, and AEMTs on scene to make sure all pertinent information is obtained and understood. Paramedics must work professionally with all other providers, as they will be looked upon as mentors and as educators who must encourage the EMR, EMT, and AEMT to keep doing the great job they do, and provide them with guidance as new medical information becomes available. The four prehospital providers all have an individual role that is linked to each of the other providers. As a paramedic, it is essential to respect and understand the training of each of the other providers so that everyone can transition care to one another seamlessly and with an awareness of the skills other providers have for the patient. Providers working within a smooth-running system build on the work done by those first on scene so that basic history taking and skills do not need to be repeated needlessly.

3. **Describe the requirements that must be met for paramedics to practice the art and science of out-of-hospital medicine.** p. 4

The education obtained in the paramedic's classroom is outstanding, and contains the most up-to-date medical information available. However, medicine is constantly changing, and often by the time books are published, information inside of them is already slowly becoming dated. For paramedics to assure themselves that they are practicing the best-practice medicine, they need to do several things. First, paramedics regularly practice high-risk, low-frequency skills such as endotracheal intubation, needle chest decompression, and surgical airways. Second, paramedics must constantly expose themselves to new medical research by obtaining continuing medical education, reading research magazines, and asking questions of physician providers. Finally, practicing paramedicine means working within a system that values regular quality assurance (QA) that establishes patient-care benchmarks that are shared with paramedics, and QA benchmarks are then used as tools to improve patient care.

4. **Describe the role of the paramedic in health care, public health, and public safety.** p. 4

As medical professionals, paramedics are respected not only by the medical community but by the public as well. This places the paramedic in an advantageous position, as paramedics have responsibilities in public health, public safety, and health care. The days where paramedics were solely responsible for prehospital care are gone. Today's paramedic must be ever vigilant and monitor for large- and small-scale public safety risks. For example, this may be accomplished by spending time at the home of an elderly couple to help them identify fall risks around the home. Paramedics also can help distinguish between serious medical conditions requiring emergency department care and less serious situations that may be triaged to a physician's office. As a patient advocate, paramedics may recognize that a patient is not taking all of his medications regularly, and by being in the home may help identify why a patient is skipping medicines. Paramedics are also constantly developing more responsibilities in areas including injury prevention, wellness visits/home health, public education, and primary care.

5. **Describe the desirable characteristics of paramedics.** pp. 4–5

Paramedics are unique in their ability to work in a vast range of environments, settings, and conditions. Thus, it's essential for paramedics to have several specific characteristics. Paramedics are flexible and open to change; they have a willingness to work in a variety of environments, and are open to taking on a challenge. As leaders, paramedics are confident, respectful, and responsible; they display good judgment, remain calm under pressure, and have the ability to think quickly and critically. Additionally, paramedics must be warm, welcoming, and friendly; patients and coworkers must feel welcome and safe around them. Further, paramedics have a drive inside of them that provides motivation, independence, and proactive thinking. In addition to the above characteristics, paramedics need to be good communicators, be open to ideas, and inspire others to do well.

6. **Explain how paramedicine has made strides toward greater recognition as a health care profession.** pp. 5–6

The original paramedics had a limited scope of care and very little freedom to practice medicine. This has drastically changed in the past 30-plus years, and today's paramedics have nearly limitless potential. Frustrated by the limited scope and poor working conditions, fragmented groups of prehospital providers began working together, first within cities, then between cities, and then across the country, to develop system-based approaches to patient care and organizational structures. Advocacy groups such as the National Association of EMTs (NAEMT) and National Registry of EMTs (NREMT) developed and began encouraging cohesiveness between organizations and created a voice to help push the paramedics education upward. Providers realized that to broaden their scope, education had to be expanded as well. As in other medical fields, the education needed to be the same between the states. This is what eventually led to the release of the 2009 national EMS education standards. All of these steps together have helped transition the role of a paramedic as a technician to that of a clinician who practices in the constantly evolving and improving field of paramedicine.

7. **List settings in which paramedics work.** pp. 6–9

Today's paramedics work in a variety of environments ranging from the ambulance and emergency departments to physician's offices and urgent care clinics. Further, the scope of paramedics has been advanced through additional training to allow specialized paramedics to work in tactical medicine, in prisons and correctional facilities, as primary care providers in remote and industrial settings as well as sports medicine, and also in critical care transport.

Case Study Review

It is important to review each emergency response you participate in as a paramedic. Similarly, we will review the case study that precedes each chapter. We will address the important points of the response as addressed by the chapter. Often, this will include the scene size-up, patient assessment, patient management, patient packaging, and transport.

Reread the case study on page 2 in Paramedic Care: Introduction to Paramedicine; *then, read the following discussion.*

This case draws attention to some of the nontraditional aspects of the new and evolving emergency medical services system.

Marcus Ward unknowingly became a classic representation of how an acute myocardial infarction can strike an individual with little warning. Generally speaking, the faster symptoms develop, the more serious an event, especially cardiac, tends to be. For Marcus, his otherwise atypical symptom of "feeling warm" rapidly progressed to his collapse. This was likely a result of his heart's electrical rhythm changing from an otherwise normal rhythm into ventricular fibrillation or ventricular tachycardia. Both of these arrhythmias are common when someone is experiencing a large myocardial infarction (MI) and should be considered signs of the MI. This is important because signs keep presenting themselves until their cause is corrected. Thus, here the arrhythmia is likely to reappear until the underlying problem (the blocked artery) is corrected. He was fortunate enough to survive because the responding health care system worked together seamlessly.

This seamless health care system began at the casino, where the security guards were likely trained as emergency medical responders (EMRs) and knew how to begin cardiopulmonary resuscitation (CPR) and use an automatic external defibrillator (AED). As is typical of a well-running system, when the EMRs were requested, 911 was simultaneously activated to quickly access advanced life support. As EMRs, the security guards quickly recognized that Marcus was not breathing and pulseless. They immediately did two important things. First, they moved Marcus a short distance to a private location. A private location prevents a crowd from forming that may impede the ability to provide optimal care and also prevents bystanders from becoming worried and anxious by Marcus's serious condition. The second important thing the EMRs did was immediately begin chest compressions and apply an AED. The most recent research tells us that when someone goes into cardiac arrest, the most important things to do are to begin chest compressions and provide early access to defibrillation. Each minute that passes without chest compressions decreases the likelihood of cardiac arrest survival by 8 to 10%.

Marcus responded immediately to the AED's first shock. The fact that the AED reported ventricular fibrillation may not mean anything to the EMR, but it is valuable information to pass to the paramedic and eventually the cardiologist. In a poorly functioning system, this information is often lost. Because Marcus began breathing immediately and opened his eyes, rescue breaths were never performed; which is OK because they may have delayed him receiving that life-saving defibrillation. However, the EMR knew that someone in cardiac arrest is oxygen deprived, and providing supplemental oxygen, most likely with a nasal cannula, helps the body recover from the event.

One of the advanced skill paramedics have is performing and interpreting the 12-lead EKG, which looks for myocardial ischemia and injury. The paramedics caring for Marcus identified anterior wall ST-segment elevation, which is seen in leads v3 and v4 on the 12-lead EKG. The anterior wall of the left ventricle receives blood via the left anterior descending artery, which in Marcus's case was occluded. Understanding the heart's anatomy allows paramedics to know that the left ventricle's lateral and septal walls could become involved as well. Time was critical for Marcus.

Again demonstrating good system function, the paramedics next did several things. They utilized their electronic transmission software in their cardiac monitor to send the 12-lead directly to an emergency department physician. The physician confirmed their findings and also activated the cardiac catheterization lab team before Marcus even arrived at the hospital. This is not possible when a system is not functioning properly.

Paramedics also began the administration of life-saving drugs that are essential in MI care. Aspirin was given, which inhibits platelets from being able to attach to other components in the clotting cascade. This prevents existing clots from getting worse. In some EMS systems, heparin may also be given, which acts on a different part of the clotting cascade, although not all paramedics routinely administer it. Nitroglycerin was given, which is a valuable tool in prehospital care. Nitroglycerin is a fast-acting vasodilator that decreases preload. When preload, or the heart's filling pressure, is decreased, the pressure within the ventricles decreases as well. With less pressure within the ventricles, the cardiac cells do not need to work as hard and thus oxygen demand goes down. With a decrease in oxygen demand, the cardiac cells do not metabolize available oxygen as quickly; EMS providers can see this manifested by the patient's chest pain/pressure decreasing. The last thing the paramedics did, and arguably the most important, was rapidly transporting Marcus to the hospital; an acute MI is one of the few times that lights and sirens transport is truly warranted.

Upon arriving at the hospital, Marcus found that the efforts of the paramedics meant that the catheterization lab team was already in the hospital. The cardiologist met Marcus in the emergency department. A very fast evaluation confirmed that Marcus was able to be moved to the catheterization lab for emergency surgery. The paramedic's 12-lead EKG had already given the cardiologist a good idea of what blood vessel in Marcus's heart was occluded. This knowledge allowed the physician to move quickly to place a catheter inside Marcus's left main coronary artery. Once there, the cardiologist could confirm the occlusion in the left anterior descending coronary artery and perform balloon angioplasty to open the blood vessel. A metal stent was placed in the artery, which helps keep another occlusion from forming in the same spot.

The moment the balloon angioplasty was performed, Marcus's emergency is over. There is no way it would have been over nearly as fast if his paramedics did not function as a key part of the health care system. His door-to-balloon time of 31 minutes was excellent—the national goal is 90 minutes. However, modern cardiac medicine also now recognizes the integral role of EMS in this and is adding EMS to the time frame and also EMS contact to balloon time with the same 90-minute goal. This integration demonstrates the ever-important role EMS has in the system approach to care.

It is important to note that following blood flow being restored through Marcus's left anterior descending coronary artery, Marcus experienced ventricular ectopy seen as premature ventricular contractions (PVCs). This is expected following reperfusion and happens because the previously oxygen-starved cardiac cells are now trying to get oxygen as quickly as they can, and this often causes ectopic beats. Following reperfusion, paramedics need to expect to see ectopic cardiac beats, including ventricular tachycardia. Although these beats may go away on their own, sometimes antidysrhythmic drugs may be required.

This is a very positive story with a great ending; Marcus gained a new appreciation for the system as a whole, and inevitably is going to help save another person's life with his purchase of an AED. Someday an EMR will likely use the AED Marcus purchased to shock a patient who is in ventricular tachycardia or ventricular fibrillation.

Content Self-Evaluation

Each of the chapters in this Workbook includes a short content review. The questions are designed to test your ability to remember what you read. At the end of this Workbook, you can find the answers to the questions as well as the pages where the topic of each question was discussed in the text. If you answered a question incorrectly or are unsure of the answer, review the pages listed.

MULTIPLE CHOICE

_____ 1. The highest level of prehospital medical care is the
   A. emergency medical responder.
   B. advanced emergency medical technician.
   C. emergency medical technician.
   D. paramedic.

_____ 2. The licensing, registering, or credentialing of a paramedic is usually provided by a state or provincial agency.
   A. True
   B. False

_____ 3. Modern EMS systems have overlapping aspects of all of the following EXCEPT
   A. health care.
   B. public politics.
   C. public health.
   D. public safety.

_____ 4. Paramedics must have many important characteristics, including
   A. strong leadership.
   B. personal insecurities.
   C. self-centeredness.
   D. personal bias.

_____ 5. How should a paramedic approach personal education?
   A. It ends with graduation from the program.
   B. A bi-annual refresher course is adequate.
   C. Actively seek out new continuing education courses.
   D. Regularly review the textbook.

_____ 6. Highly functioning paramedics recognize that rarely performed skills
   A. don't need to be practiced.
   B. require regular practice.
   C. are likely unnecessary.
   D. are unlikely to benefit patients.

_____ 7. The primary focus of the EMR is to
   A. initiate lifesaving interventions.
   B. differentiate between stable and critical patients.
   C. diagnose underlying medical conditions.
   D. begin some advanced procedures.

_____ 8. The effect of the 2009 National EMS education standards was to
   A. limit the paramedics scope of care.
   B. restrict progressive EMS systems.
   C. raise the educational bar.
   D. reduce the total classroom hours.

_____ 9. One of the greatest advances in the paramedicine field was the introduction of
   A. prehospital medical research.
   B. nurses into ambulances.
   C. EMS unions.
   D. standardized billing practices.

_____ 10. An example of expanding a paramedic's scope of practice includes training to
   A. perform emergency caesarean sections.
   B. monitor an intra-aortic balloon pump.
   C. use tasers to calm patients.
   D. insert ICP monitors.

_____ 11. Paramedics working in emergency departments (EDs) would be expected to
   A. take over the nursing role.
   B. work alongside a registered nurse.
   C. replace other advanced providers.
   D. be responsible for the entire ED.

_____ 12. Typically, paramedics are licensed and/or credentialed by their
   A. local governing body.
   B. individual agency.
   C. state/provincial government.
   D. federal government.

_____ 13. As the role of paramedics expands, they may be expected to be
   A. public educators.
   B. injury prevention advocates.
   C. public safety officers.
   D. patient advocates.
   E. all of the above.

_____ **14.** The best-practice medicine performed in today's EMS systems is based on
  A. anecdotes.
  B. traditional medical care.
  C. physician personal preferences.
  D. EMS-based medical research.

_____ **15.** Paramedics see an expanded scope of practice when moving into which of the following fields?
  A. Critical care transport
  B. Primary care
  C. Industrial medicine
  D. Sports medicine
  E. All of the above

LISTING

16. List the major ways in which the 2009 national EMS education standards have raised the education of paramedics to a higher level.

_____
_____
_____
_____
_____

17. List the additional training associated with the following areas of the paramedic's expanded scope of practice.

A. Critical care transport

_____
_____

B. Industrial medicine

_____
_____

C. Sports medicine

_____
_____

©2013 Pearson Education, Inc.
Paramedic Care: Principles & Practice, Vol. 1, 4th Ed.

EMS Systems

Review of Chapter Objectives

After reading this chapter, you should be able to:

1. **Define key terms introduced in this chapter.**

   Knowing and being able to apply the key terms in each chapter is critical to understanding chapter concepts. Write the list of key terms. Then write the definition of each one in your own words. Check your understanding by confirming the definitions in the text glossary. Correct any misunderstandings. Create a study aid by writing each key term on the front of an index card and the definition on the back. Use the cards to quiz yourself or to have someone quiz you.

2. **Describe the out-of-hospital and in-hospital components of EMS systems.** p. 14

   The emergency medical system is a network of people who initiate the delivery of emergency medical care and then continue that care through the hospital and even after patient discharge. EMTs and paramedics are a piece of this network that incorporates many groups of people both outside of and inside of the hospital. Each component of the system is required for the system itself to function effectively. Paramedics have an ability to function in both out-of-hospital and in-hospital components, which makes it even more important that paramedics understand how system components integrate with one another and how failure of one component can affect the entire system.

   Out of-hospital system components include:

   - Members of the community who are trained in first aid and CPR and know how and when to access the EMS system
   - Communication systems to create public access for emergency medical dispatch and reliable communication between EMS agencies and the 911 centers
   - EMS providers, including the EMR, EMT, AEMT, and paramedic
   - Fire/rescue and hazardous-material services
   - Law enforcement
   - Public utilities, including power and gas companies and road workers
   - Resource centers, including poison control and outreach clinics

   In-hospital system components include:

   - Emergency department nurses
   - Mid-level medical practitioners, including physician assistants and advance-practice nurses
   - Emergency department physicians
   - Ancillary services such as radiology, respiratory therapy, and spiritual services
   - Specialty physicians such as trauma surgeons, cardiologists, and neurosurgeons
   - Social workers
   - Mental health providers
   - Rehabilitation services

3. Given various scenarios, explain how EMS systems work to respond to out-of-hospital emergencies. p. 14

Henry is 64 years old, in good health, and sees his doctor regularly. One day, while Henry was treating his three grandchildren to lunch, he, without warning, dropped his spoon and slumped to the side. His waiter, having recently been trained in first aid, immediately asked if he was alright, and Henry could only mumble nonsense words while his right arm sat limp to his side. With her first aid training, the sever recognized that Henry could be having a stroke, and 911 was called within 3 minutes. Once 911 was activated, an emergency medical dispatcher, through prearrival instructions, confirmed Henry was awake and breathing and also confirmed the restaurant's address, while a second dispatcher used the computer-aided dispatch program to dispatch the closest BLS rescue squad and ALS ambulance to the scene. First responders arrived within 4 minutes of the 911 call and the ambulance arrived 3 minutes later. By the time Henry's paramedics walked in, the BLS crew had applied oxygen to Henry with a nasal cannula, had obtained his vital signs, and reported to the paramedics that Henry had positive findings on the Cincinnati Stroke Scale.

When the paramedics took over Henry's care, they only had to ask a few questions, because the EMTs were able to provide Henry's medicines, allergies, past medical history, and the onset of his symptoms. Henry was prepared for transport in the ambulance 10 minutes after the ambulance arrived. During transport the paramedics established intravenous access, repeated vital signs, and performed a fibrinolytic checklist. The closest emergency department was bypassed because the paramedics knew that their system had a designated primary stroke center an extra 10 minutes away. They radioed in a "Code Stroke," and upon their arrival at the hospital, Henry was met in the emergency department (ED) with not only an ED physician, but also the members of the hospitals stroke team, which included a neurologist.

Henry was taken directly to a CT scanner, where a radiologist confirmed that Henry was not bleeding inside of his head. After he was brought back to the emergency department, the ED physician confirmed the paramedic's fibrinolytic checklist findings and determined that Henry was a candidate for the fibrinolytics, which he received less than 50 minutes after his symptoms began. During the rest of his hospitalization, Henry's care was supervised by the neurologist. After four days in the hospital, Henry had nearly full strength in his right arm and leg and could speak with only a hint of slurring in his words. He was discharged and prescribed a month of rehabilitation therapy with the hospital's stroke rehabilitation team. Henry had such a positive outcome because the entire EMS system had been set up, from initial emergency through rehabilitation.

4. Link key events in the history of EMS to the development of the modern EMS system. pp. 15–22

There is a long history of individuals providing care in the out-of-hospital setting, beginning in ancient times. The cardinal events in the history of EMS include the first organized use of patient transport (and the ambulance) by Jean Larrey, chief surgeon for Napoleon. Although simply a horse-drawn cart called an *ambulance volante* (flying ambulance), it represented the first recognized attempt to bring the injured from the field to medical care. Wars continued to be the impetus to improve out-of-hospital care. The American Civil War, World Wars I and II, and the Korean and Vietnamese conflicts all brought substantial changes to field care and transport. The war in Vietnam saw a greater reduction in mortality associated with immediate care in the field and rapid access to surgery than was the case in any previous conflict.

However, the single greatest event in the development of modern-day EMS was the National Highway Safety Act of 1966. This act, for the first time and on a national level, recognized emergency medical services and financially supported their development. Under that act, and its establishment of the Department of Transportation (DOT) as overseeing agency, the nation soon had the first national EMS training curriculum, new criteria for ambulance design (the KKK specifications), and the creation of state-led agencies to coordinate EMS development. Later federal legislation created EMS systems through the guidance of the Department of Health, Education, and Welfare, and since then several federal initiatives have continued to improve the nation's EMS system, mostly under the leadership of the DOT.

The twenty-first century has brought about great change in today's EMS systems. The National Scope of Practice model defines those skills expected of the Emergency Medical Responder (EMR), the Emergency Medical Technician (EMT), the Advanced Emergency Medical Technician (AEMT), and the paramedic. The new educational standards describe the competencies expected of these levels of providers and change the face of EMS classrooms. Documents developed by the National Academies of Science (*At the Crossroads*) and the American College of Emergency Physicians (*National Report Card*) identify where improvements in our system are required. These efforts continue to evolve the emergency medical services system. The largest single event causing system change was the terrorist attacks on September 11, 2001. In the wake of these attacks, the weaknesses in EMS system response were identified. In response to this, the National Incident Management System (NIMS) was created and charged with standardizing response to major incidents. Also in 2001, Medicare and Medicaid billing practices were changed, allowing for increased cost recuperation for EMS helicopters; this has led to a tripling in the fleet of EMS helicopters.

5. **Describe each of the ten components of EMS systems according to the Statewide EMS Technical Assessment Program.** p. 19

NHTSA has defined the following components for EMS systems:

- **Regulation and policy**—Each state must have laws, regulations, policies, and procedures that govern its EMS system.
- **Resources management**—Each state must have central control of health care resources to ensure that all patients have equal access to emergency care.
- **Human resources and training**—Each state must require that all EMS providers are taught by qualified instructors using a standardized curriculum.
- **Transportation**—Each state must ensure that patients are safely and reliably transported by ground or air ambulance.
- **Facilities**—Each state must ensure that every seriously ill or injured patient is delivered to an appropriate medical facility in a timely manner.
- **Communications**—Each state must have a system for public access to EMS along with communications among dispatchers, ambulance crews, and hospital personnel.
- **Trauma systems**—Each state should develop a system of specialized care for trauma patients, including the designation of trauma centers and systems to ensure patients arrive at the appropriate facility in a timely manner.
- **Public information and education**—EMS personnel should participate in programs designed to educate the public in injury prevention, emergency recognition, system access, and first aid.
- **Medical direction**—Each EMS system must have a physician medical director responsible for delegating medical practice to prehospital care providers and overseeing patient care.
- **Evaluation**—Each state must have a quality improvement system for continuing evaluation and upgrading of the EMS system.

6. **Discuss the vision and documents that are guiding EMS into the future.** pp. 20-22

Three major papers are pushing EMS forward: *EMS Agenda for the Future* published in 1996 by the National Highway Traffic Safety Administration (NHTSA), *Emergency Medical Services: At the Crossroads* published in 2006 by the National Academies Institute of Medicine, and *The National Report Card on the State of Emergency Medicine: Evaluating the Environment of Emergency Care Systems State by State* released by the American College of Emergency Physicians (ACEP) in 2006.

EMS Agenda for the Future views the future of EMS as integrated in community-based health care management. In the paper's view, EMS will grow into a part of the system where providers provide injury and illness prevention, acute care management, and also help provide post-event follow-up to aid in the management of long-term illnesses. The goal of this vision is to help alleviate stresses on primary care physicians as well as emergency departments. To achieve this vision, EMS must accomplish 14 attributes:

- Integration of health services
- EMS research
- Legislation and regulation
- System finance
- Human resources

- Medical direction
- Education systems
- Public education
- Prevention
- Public access
- Communication systems
- Clinical care
- Information systems
- Evaluation

A full decade later, *Emergency Medical Services: At the Crossroads* became a bold statement in the reality of how poorly systems of the time were functioning. Although many great advances have been made, there are gaping holes in how EMS systems are functioning across the nation. The authors found many problems at the federal level and specified several key areas needing improvement in government leadership, system organization, and quality assurance and medical care standardization.

Finally, *The National Report Card on the State of Emergency Medicine: Evaluating the Environment of Emergency Care Systems State by State* emphasized that the problems in emergency medicine are not isolated to EMS systems; rather, the problems are spread across hospital emergency departments. The most important piece of this paper was that it demonstrated that although both EMS and hospitals have major problems in their care, the problems are intimately linked and must be addressed together. The impact of this paper was that it brought to the forefront the need for health care systems to acknowledge EMS as an important link in the health care system and that the needs of all must be corrected together.

7. **Discuss the contemporary problems facing EMS as described in the Institute of Medicine document *Emergency Medical Services: At the Crossroads.***

p. 21

The fragmented structure of the country's emergency and trauma care was broken apart in *Emergency Medical Services: At the Crossroads.* Among the many system weaknesses identified, it found that there is a lack of national coordination; EMS, fire, and public safety are fragmented and in many regions in the United States they cannot easily communicate between agencies. Within given regions, EMS doesn't consistently transport patients to appropriate destinations, resulting in suboptimal patient care, which is also exacerbated by ineffective communication between EMS agencies and the hospitals. When responding to emergencies, response times are measured differently. Times may begin as early as the initial 911 call or start as late as when a vehicle begins responding.

On the arrival end, some time measurements end when the first vehicle arrives on scene, whereas others do not end until crews arrive at the patient's side. Another concern identified is that EMS quality is not measured in the same manner between programs and across the states. Quality assurance programs exist; however, success measurements are not consistent. Despite the attacks in 2001 and the major hurricanes since, many EMS systems are not prepared for the patient surges seen during a disaster. At the same time, providers within systems are also not trained in responses to natural and human-caused disasters. The paper also highlighted that there is no single EMS identity. The authors found that police and fire receive more respect and recognition than EMS providers as public safety officers, whereas physicians and nurses have more respect in the health care profession. Because EMS affiliates closely with both—the public safety and health care groups—a unique identity must be found so that education, salaries, and work conditions can improve. Finally, the *Emergency Medical Services: At the Crossroads* paper demonstrated that there is a lack of evidence-based medicine in EMS and highlighted the need for improved and ongoing EMS research.

8. **Give examples of various approaches to and configurations of EMS systems in the United States.**

p. 22

The structure of today's EMS systems varies across the country. One structure is the fire-based system, where ambulances are operated by and structured underneath the fire services. Third-service systems are government systems separate from fire or police and are generally independent, government-based organizations. Many cities rely on private ambulance services, which run independently with limited government oversight. These private services may be nonprofit or for-profit companies. Hospital-based systems exist in many regions, where the major hospital or health care system provides oversight and owns the EMS system. Volunteer services provide EMS system care for the majority of the geographic area of the United States and may be private nonprofit organizations or public nonprofit organizations. Finally, hybrid organizations are a combination of any two or more of these groups.

9. **Explain the role of EMS in the chain of survival from cardiac arrest and in the optimal care of all emergency patients.** **p. 22**

The American Heart Association coined the phrase "the chain of survival" to highlight the importance of early recognition and management of patients in cardiac arrest. Originally, there were four links in the chain of survival: immediate recognition and access to 911, early CPR, rapid defibrillation, and early advanced cardiac life support (ACLS). However, today's chain has fifth link added: integrated post–cardiac arrest care. EMS plays a vital link in this chain of survival. Even with bystander recognition of cardiac arrest and their prompt calling of 911, emergency medical services must rapidly respond with the appropriate resources. Paramedics bring ACLS to the patient; however, the best ACLS in the world is useless if the public is not properly trained to rapidly recognize patients in cardiac arrest and begin CPR while calling 911. When patients are successfully resuscitated, many post–cardiac arrest interventions become important, including careful blood pressure management and therapeutic hypothermia. The sooner these begin the better, and EMS not only has the tools to begin these interventions, but there is actually research that shows if EMS providers do not provide these interventions or make sure patients are taken to hospitals capable of continuing these interventions, then the odds of patient survival decline.

The cardiac arrest chain of survival is only one example of how EMS providers are only one, but a very important, link in many survival chains. Paramedics and EMS systems are vital links in the survival chains for patients experiencing acute strokes, major trauma, sepsis (a systemic infection), and seizures.

10. **Describe the purposes of the national documents guiding EMS education and practice.** **p. 23**

Originally when EMTs and paramedics were educated, the content of that education was largely determined by local governing bodies and a given education institution. This led to the fragmenting of the EMS system on a national scale because EMTs and paramedics across the country ended up with drastically different capabilities, education, and scopes of practice.

To address this problem, the NHTSA published the *National EMS Core Content* (2005), which highlighted the skills EMS professionals should have. Closely following this paper was the *National EMS Scope of Practice* (2005), which defined the roles of different level EMS providers by what skills they each should be able to perform. This paper not only generated consistency across EMS systems, but also increased the bar for EMS classroom education. By creating consistent scopes of practice for EMS providers, education within different EMS systems is more easily standardized. Finally, the release of the *National EMS Instructional Guidelines* presented a consistent standardization of the information and skills taught within EMS classrooms while increasing latitude for EMS instructors to determine how they would like to present that information.

11. **Discuss typical components of local- and state-level EMS systems.** **p. 23**

Local EMS systems are typically associated with given municipalities and/or counties. These local systems establish administrative oversight and are responsible for local resources, medical protocols, and performance standards and guidelines. The oversight for these systems is most often through a planning board that consists of representatives from agencies and groups with a stake in the EMS system. These groups are typically community/government representatives, emergency department physicians, nursing associations, fire and police departments, as well as "consumers" or laypersons from the region. In addition to general oversight, the planning board also typically defines the qualifications to work within the EMS system, defines the quality assurance system, and establishes measures for assuring system readiness and performance.

The state-level EMS system provides a more generalized influence on the local-level EMS systems. Some of the responsibilities of state systems include funding and legislation. The state system determines licensing requirements and certifies or licenses individuals to practice within the state. Other state-level activities are the development of EMS regulations, state-wide quality assurance, and the creation of regional EMS advisory councils/systems. EMS is truly systems within systems. There is a national EMS system, a state EMS system, a regional EMS system, and finally the local EMS system.

12. Explain the purpose and responsibilities of physician medical directors in EMS services. p. 23

The medical director is a physician who is legally responsible for all clinical and patient-care aspects of an EMS system. Prehospital care provided by the paramedic or other EMS personnel is provided under the license of the medical director, regardless of who their employer is.

A paramedic functions only under the supervision and direction of a medical direction physician. That oversight is provided as either on-line medical direction or off-line medical direction. Off-line medical direction involves the physician's participation in personnel and equipment selection, training, protocol development, quality improvement, and acting as an EMS and patient advocate within the health profession. On-line medical direction consists of direct radio or phone consultation and oversight of paramedics and other prehospital care providers while they are caring for a patient. The ultimate responsibility for all care offered by the paramedic rests with the medical direction physician.

13. Give examples of on-line medical direction and off-line medical oversight. pp. 23–24

Both on-line and off-line medical direction provide medical supervision of the EMS system and prehospital and out-of-hospital patient care. Off-line medical oversight allows paramedics the opportunity to practice "prehospital medicine" under the license and supervision of the medical director, including use of established protocols, standing orders, and algorithms developed by the medical director. On-line medical direction provides access to direct medical consultation for EMS personnel during the care of the emergency patient when the best approach to a patient's care may not be very clear or is particularly challenging.

14. Describe the purposes of the National Registry of EMTs and the several professional organizations in EMS. p. 28

National associations identify standards for performance in EMS and advocate for patient care and the professional stature of their members. The National Registry of EMTs maintains a national standard, through testing, at the Emergency Medical Technician, Advanced Emergency Medical Technician, and paramedic levels of EMS training. Other standard-setting agencies establish the criteria and standards for system performance. For example, the Joint Committee on Educational Programs for the Paramedic sets standards for institutions educating paramedics. The American Heart Association sets standards for basic and advanced cardiac life support. The American College of Emergency Physicians recommends a list of ALS equipment for ambulances. The American College of Surgeons establishes a listing of essential BLS ambulance equipment.

15. Recognize professional journals related to the practice of EMS. p. 28

Professional journals serve as an outlet for publishing EMS-related research as well as a means for communicating major events and medical practice changes on a national level. Many journals also contain continuing medical education, national employment opportunities, and tips and strategies for improving your personal and system performance. Among these journals are the following:

- *Academic Emergency Medicine*
- *American Journal of Emergency Medicine*
- *Annals of Emergency Medicine*
- *EMS World Magazine*
- *Journal of Emergency Medical Services*
- *Journal of Pediatric Emergency Medicine*
- *Journal of Trauma: Injury, Infection, and Critical Care*
- *Prehospital Emergency Care*

Although this is not a complete list, these journals are examples of those that discuss or are devoted to prehospital care. Of particular note, *Prehospital Emergency Care* is the only journal that is dedicated to only publishing 100% peer-reviewed medical research articles on topics specific to out-of-hospital medical care.

16. Describe the intent of the General Services Administration KKK-A-1822 Federal Specifications for Ambulances. p. 30

The goal for establishing the KKK-A-1822 Federal Specifications for Ambulances was to standardize ambulance design to optimize and permit life-sustaining interventions during transport to definitive care facilities. Three different types of ambulances were defined in KKK-A-1822: Type I, Type II, and Type III ambulances. In addition to specifying ambulance types, the KKK-A-1822 established that only registered ambulances may display the Star of Life symbol and stated that registered ambulances must have the word *Ambulance* in mirror image on the front of the vehicle. These rules helped develop a standardized shape and presentation of ambulances across the country for easy recognition.

Over the years, KKK-A-1822 has undergone four revisions to improve patient and provider safety. These revisions established internal noise protection standards, modernized lighting requirements, reduced vehicle roll risk by widening the axles, improved ventilation systems, improved patient and provider safety systems, and, in 2007, the most noticeable modern change required new ambulances to have a standardized paint pattern on the back of ambulances to improve roadside safety.

17. Describe the purpose for categorizing receiving hospital facilities by their capabilities. pp. 30–31

Hospitals across the country vary greatly in their capability to manage specialized patient groups, particularly those requiring emergent intervention in life-threatening situations, including trauma, heart attacks, and strokes. National standards have been developed to allow hospitals to be designated for emergent and long-term management of these specialized patients based on their physician and allied professional readiness, surgical suite readiness, and rehabilitation capabilities. When a hospital obtains designation as a specialized service center such as trauma center, primary stroke center, children's hospital, or chest pain center, it is a sign not only to the public but also to EMS systems of their advanced readiness.

For the purposes of EMS systems, hospital designations are important. Hospitals with designations can more rapidly manage those specific patient groups. It is a signal for transporting ambulances that patients can be more appropriately treated at designated hospitals than at a local hospital without those resources. This means that ambulances may bypass the closest hospital for one farther away that is designated to treat the patient being transported. EMS providers need to triage and transport patients to specialized hospitals when they are available to help ensure the best care for patients.

18. Explain the purpose and components of an effective continuous quality improvement program. pp. 31–32

Continuous quality improvement (CQI) is an ongoing effort to refine and improve the system to ensure the highest level of service possible. It involves six basic components: identifying system-wide problems, elaborating on the probable causes, listing solutions, outlining a plan of corrective action, providing resources and support to ensure success, and reevaluating the results and system performance continuously. CQI system review uses positive reinforcement and support to identify and improve patient care. It can identify areas for improvement and ways to allocate resources to make those improvements, frequently through continuing medical education. When questions arise about the benefits of care offered by a system, a CQI program can suggest research projects to investigate the real value of procedures, equipment, and protocols. The real key to effective CQI is the positive and reinforcing nature of its approach to system improvement.

19. Describe how you can contribute to greater patient safety in emergency medical services. pp. 33–34

Medical errors need to be acknowledged as part of medicine; however, they do not need to be accepted. It is important to acknowledge they exist so that we can identify and minimize how they occur.

The three major causes for medical errors are skill-based failures, rules-based failures, and knowledge-based failures. EMS can do a lot to minimize errors in these areas by identifying low-volume and high-risk skills and practicing them regularly; following rules designed to ensure provider and patient safety, such as requiring patients to always be transported with safety belts secured; and by constantly reviewing the medical literature to stay current on best-practice medicine.

In addition, there are several high-risk areas for EMS-related medical errors. Particular focus needs to be given to proper communication and safety during these times. Communication errors between family and hospitals, particularly when handing off a patient from one EMS service to another, or at the hospital, can allow for information pertinent to the patient's complaint, history, allergies, or field-administered medicines to be missed. Medication administration is another area at high risk for error. Strive to always ensure administration of the proper drug and dose. It is also erroneous to fail to administer a needed medicine.

Airway management is an area filled with high-risk situations, and is the focus of national attention and research. Prehospital providers need to be diligent about proper and aggressive airway management, and paramedics must always remain competent on advanced airway skills, especially intubation.

Other times of high risk for patient injury include: patient drops, ambulance crashes, spinal immobilization, and resuscitation termination. Be diligent in making sure to put patient safety first and remain familiar with safety strategies and proper techniques when performing skills. Injuring or killing a patient can easily end a paramedic's career.

20. Explain the role of research in EMS. pp. 34–35

Research is essential in ensuring that the equipment and procedures used in the out-of-hospital setting are safe, benefit the patient, and are worth any potential risks of employing them. Research attempts to objectively evaluate the performance of interventions in an unbiased way. Research is a process that involves asking a question (stating a hypothesis), investigating any existing research, designing a study that is unbiased and fairly measures performance, collecting and analyzing data, assessing and evaluating results against the hypothesis, and reporting the findings. Evidence-based medicine (EBM) evaluates research to determine which procedures in emergency medicine have a positive impact on patient outcome and which do not. This process may cause us to reevaluate the tools and procedures that were once considered standard in prehospital care.

Case Study Review

Reread the case study on pages 13 and 14 in Paramedic Care: Introduction to Paramedicine; *then, read the following discussion.*

This case study demonstrates the coming together of personnel from many agencies to meet the prehospital needs of a patient—an EMS system.

The case study highlights the different facets of EMS response. Observing the crash, you recognize the need for a response and access the system by using a cell phone to dial the universal entry number 911. The initial dispatcher quickly directs your call to the EMS area dispatcher, and the dispatcher starts numerous agencies en route to the scene—the fire department (BLS), the rescue service, and an ALS ambulance. The police are also notified and begin their response. The dispatcher gathers further information about the crash to update the responding personnel and possibly modify the response. Once on the scene, the BLS providers assume patient-care responsibilities by ensuring that the scene is safe, analyzing the mechanism of injury, and taking information from you. From this information and the results of a quick physical assessment (the initial assessment) of the patients, they triage the patients and call the dispatcher for an additional ALS ambulance and air medical transport.

An additional arriving fire unit further ensures traffic control and scene safety and establishes a landing zone. The highest-trained EMS care provider assumes overall patient-care coordination responsibilities. He calls for the patients to be distributed to the most appropriate facilities, ensuring that the patients receive the best of care and that no single facility is overloaded by the arrival of patients. This process, as established by the medical direction system and supervised by a resource hospital, also ensures that the most appropriate hospital resources are used for the most seriously injured patients. Patients are moved quickly to the appropriate facilities. The child is rushed by air to the pediatric trauma center, while the adults are rushed to other appropriate trauma centers. In this case study, various providers from various services work together efficiently to ensure that patients are removed from the crash scene quickly. This study is thus an excellent example of an EMS system operating as it should.

What is not mentioned here is that the care given by the providers is well coordinated because the various services practice working together in disaster drills and because continuous quality improvement programs have identified system weaknesses and have taken corrective action before these patients were placed in need. Ongoing education and skills maintenance exercises keep the providers current in skills and knowledge. Finally, the system's CQI committee will review this response, identify strengths, and correct any weaknesses it reveals through education and revised protocols. Again, these are signs of a healthy EMS system.

Content Self-Evaluation

MULTIPLE CHOICE

_____ 1. An Emergency Medical Services system is a network of personnel, equipment, and resources established to deliver aid and emergency care to the community.
   A. True
   B. False

_____ 2. The date of the earliest recorded medical care procedures is
   A. about 5,000 years ago.   D. 1562.
   B. about 2,000 years ago.   E. 1666.
   C. 1497.

_____ 3. In a well-developed EMS system, trained first responders are likely to be
   A. police officers.   D. teachers.
   B. firefighters.   E. all of the above.
   C. lifeguards.

_____ 4. In a non-tiered EMS system, in which order do care providers have contact with the patient?
   A. Emergency physician, dispatcher, ALS provider, BLS provider
   B. Dispatcher, ALS provider or BLS provider, emergency physician
   C. Dispatcher, BLS provider, ALS provider, emergency physician
   D. Dispatcher, BLS provider, emergency physician, ALS provider
   E. None of the above

_____ 5. The advent of the ambulance is generally credited to
   A. Napoleon in 1812.   D. Cincinnati, Ohio, in 1865.
   B. Jean Larrey in 1797.   E. Bellevue Hospital in 1869.
   C. Clara Barton in 1862.

_____ 6. A report focusing on the problem of accidental death and legislation that began modern-day EMS dates to
   A. 1950.   D. 1981.
   B. 1966.   E. 1988.
   C. 1972.

_____ 7. Which of the following was NOT a component of the Emergency Medical Services Systems Act of 1973?
   A. Communications   D. Access to care
   B. System financing   E. System evaluation
   C. Training

_____ 8. The medical director is a physician who is legally responsible for all patient care offered by the system he oversees.
   A. True
   B. False

_____ 9. The intervener physician is a physician who is
   A. not affiliated with the system of medical direction.
   B. at the scene of an emergency.
   C. a trained emergency physician.
   D. both A and B.
   E. none of the above.

_____ 10. When on-line medical direction is established and an intervener physician is present, is willing to accept patient-care responsibility, performs interventions consistent with the system protocols, and agrees to document the interventions as required by the system, the paramedic should
   A. relinquish patient-care responsibilities.
   B. retain patient-care authority.
   C. relinquish patient-care responsibilities only if the physician agrees to ride to the hospital.
   D. retain patient-care responsibilities in cases of physician disagreement.
   E. none of the above.

_____ 11. Off-line medical direction includes which of the following?
   A. Protocols   D. Quality assurance
   B. Training guidelines   E. All of the above
   C. Personnel selection policies

_____ 12. Which of the following is NOT one of the four "Ts" of emergency care?
   A. Triage   D. Transport
   B. Transfer   E. Treatment
   C. Termination of care

_____ 13. Which of the following statements is NOT true?
   A. The ability to recognize cardiac emergencies can save lives.
   B. Over 300,000 cardiac arrests per year occur before the patient reaches the hospital.
   C. Most cardiac arrests happen immediately upon onset of symptoms.
   D. If bystanders or the patient call in time, many cardiac arrests can be prevented.
   E. All of the above are NOT true.

_____ 14. Current research shows that placing automatic defibrillators in public places is reducing cardiac arrest mortality.
   A. True
   B. False

_____ 15. Multiple community phone numbers for citizen access to emergency medical services will
   A. ensure efficient system entry.
   B. add minutes to system entry.
   C. ensure callback capability.
   D. ensure instant routing to the proper agency.
   E. all of the above.

_____ 16. There are great disadvantages to dispatching EMS, fire, and police from a single control center.
   A. True
   B. False

_____ 17. The dispatch system that provides caller interrogation, predetermined response configurations, and prearrival instructions is
   A. system status management.   D. caller interrogation.
   B. enhanced 911.   E. none of the above.
   C. priority dispatch.

©2013 Pearson Education, Inc.
Paramedic Care: Principles & Practice, Vol. 1, 4th Ed.

_____ **18.** There may be some increased liability for a system providing prearrival instructions.
  A. True
  B. False

_____ **19.** The goal of dispatch and response in an effective EMS is to have
  A. AEDs on the scene within 4 minutes.
  B. ALS units on the scene within 4 minutes.
  C. CPR initiated within 4 minutes of cardiac arrest.
  D. all of the above.
  E. none of the above.

_____ **20.** The learning domain associated with skills is
  A. cognitive.
  B. psychomotor.
  C. affective.
  D. didactic.
  E. dexterous.

_____ **21.** The process by which a state or other governmental agency grants permission to engage in a given occupation is
  A. licensure.
  B. certification.
  C. registration.
  D. reciprocity.
  E. tenure.

_____ **22.** Granting someone recognition for meeting the qualifications of another agency is called
  A. licensure.
  B. certification.
  C. registration.
  D. reciprocity.
  E. tenure.

_____ **23.** Which association administers a standardized test for all EMS provider levels and serves as the national standard for certification competency?
  A. National Association of EMTs
  B. National Registry of EMTs
  C. National Association of EMS Educators
  D. National Association of EMS Physicians
  E. National EMS Management Association

_____ **24.** What are some of the benefits to regularly reading EMS-related magazines and journals?
  A. Receive continuing education
  B. Career advancement opportunities
  C. Review current research publications
  D. Identify new skill techniques
  E. All of the above

_____ **25.** Which paper was updated in 2002 to establish guidelines improving patient and provider safety during transport?
  A. _EMS Agenda for the Future_
  B. _National EMS Core Content_
  C. KKK-A-1822
  D. _EMS at the Crossroads_
  E. EMS Agenda for the Future

_____ **26.** _EMS Agenda for the Future_ brought what idea to the forefront for EMS systems?
  A. EMS systems are fragmented across the United States.
  B. EMS has an integral role in the overall health care system.
  C. There is no consistent education for EMS providers nationally.
  D. There is no role in public health for EMS providers.
  E. A national standard for EMS education is needed.

_____ **27.** The body that sets accreditation standards for paramedic education programs is the
  A. Committee on Accreditation of Educational Programs for the EMS Professions.
  B. National Association of EMTs.
  C. National Registry of EMTs.
  D. National Council of State EMS Training Coordinators.
  E. American College of Emergency Physicians.

28. In the chain of survival, which group's patient care is most important for patient survival?
- **A.** Bystanders
- **B.** First responders
- **C.** Paramedics
- **D.** Physicians
- **E.** All of the above

29. The agency responsible for establishing criteria for the design of ambulances is the
- **A.** American College of Surgeons.
- **B.** American College of Emergency Physicians.
- **C.** U.S. General Services Administration.
- **D.** U.S. Military Assistance to Traffic and Safety Group.
- **E.** National Association of EMTs.

30. A standard van with a raised roof that is configured as an ambulance is categorized as which type of ambulance?
- **A.** Type I
- **B.** Type II
- **C.** Type III
- **D.** Type A
- **E.** Type B

31. Development of EMS regulations and statutes is performed by
- **A.** local EMS systems.
- **B.** regional advisory councils.
- **C.** state EMS agencies.
- **D.** federal EMS agencies.
- **E.** the U.S. Department of Transportation.

32. A hospital designated as a receiving facility for the EMS system should have which of the following?
- **A.** An emergency department
- **B.** 24-hour emergency physician coverage
- **C.** Surgical facilities and coverage
- **D.** Critical and intensive care units
- **E.** All of the above

33. Which of the following is NOT a part of a well-designed disaster plan?
- **A.** Mutual aid agreements among neighboring municipalities, services, and systems
- **B.** A rigid communications system
- **C.** Frequent disaster plan tests and drills
- **D.** Integration of all system components
- **E.** A coordinated central management agency

34. A major complaint regarding quality assurance programs is that they tend to
- **A.** be one-time efforts.
- **B.** address only procedural issues.
- **C.** be punitive in nature.
- **D.** not examine protocol issues.
- **E.** create divisions among care workers on staff.

35. Continuous quality improvement differs from quality assurance in that it
- **A.** emphasizes customer satisfaction.
- **B.** rewards or reinforces good behavior.
- **C.** examines billing practices.
- **D.** evaluates maintenance activities.
- **E.** all the above.

36. Which of the following is NOT one of the standard rules of evidence used to evaluate a proposed change in the EMS system?
- **A.** There must be a basis for change.
- **B.** The old procedure must be deemed no longer medically acceptable.
- **C.** The change must be clinically important.

D. The change must be affordable, practical, and teachable.

E. None of the above is standard rule of evidence.

_____ 37. Ethics are best defined as

A. protocols and policies for conduct.

B. rules or standards governing the performance of a profession.

C. legal principles governing potential lawsuits.

D. the four elements needed to determine negligence.

E. justifications for actions.

_____ 38. To the patient, it may be more important to receive care from a provider who seems to be interested in him and empathetic than to receive the most technically correct care.

A. True

B. False

_____ 39. Difficulty in which aspect of care can result in errors in patient care?

A. Communication

B. Medication administration

C. Airway management

D. Spinal immobilization

E. All of the above

_____ 40. EMS research should answer which question?

A. What prehospital interventions decrease mortality?

B. What skills can be safely performed by paramedics?

C. What strategies gather the largest profit margin?

D. Are paramedics truly needed?

E. Should nurses serve in EMS?

LISTING

Identify the agency or association most closely linked with the following guidelines or papers for EMS:

41. National standard curricula for EMS provider _____

_____

42. Criteria for ambulance design _____

_____

43. National standard for EMS certification and testing _____

_____

44. *Emergency Medical Services: At the Crossroads* _____

_____

45. Criteria for paramedic education programs _____

_____

Special Project

The EMS Agenda for the Future

A. Describe the purpose of the *EMS Agenda for the Future*.

_____

_____

_____

_____

_____

_____

_____

_____

_____

_____

_____

_____

_____

_____

B. List at least six of the EMS attributes defined by the *EMS Agenda for the Future*.

_____

_____

_____

_____

_____

_____

_____

_____

©2013 Pearson Education, Inc.
Paramedic Care: Principles & Practice, Vol. 1, 4th Ed.

3

Roles and Responsibilities of the Paramedic

Review of Chapter Objectives

After reading this chapter, you should be able to:

1. **Define key terms introduced in this chapter.**

   Knowing and being able to apply the key terms in each chapter is critical to understanding chapter concepts. Write the list of key terms. Then write the definition of each one in your own words. Check your understanding by confirming the definitions in the text glossary. Correct any misunderstandings. Create a study aid by writing each key term on the front of an index card and the definition on the back. Use the cards to quiz yourself or to have someone quiz you.

2. **Discuss each of the primary responsibilities of paramedics.**   pp. 41–46

   The primary duties of paramedics extend well beyond direct patient care and include:

   - **Preparation**—Paramedics must be mentally, physically, and emotionally ready to respond to any call; know local protocols, geography, and equipment; and ensure that the vehicle and equipment are all in proper working order.
   - **Response**—Paramedics must drive responsibly, ensuring a timely yet safe response, always operating emergency vehicles with due regard. It is also essential to confirm the response address and also anticipate the need for other emergency services early.
   - **Scene size-up**—Paramedics must assess the scene to determine the safety of the scene, including identification of any hazards and the need for Standard Precautions, the number of ill or injured, the need for any additional resources, and the mechanism of injury or the nature of the illness. Scene safety is of the utmost importance; never enter a scene that is not safe.
   - **Patient assessment**—Once at the patient's side, the paramedic must determine whether or not the patient needs cervical immobilization as well as his level of consciousness and the stability of the airway, breathing, and circulation. Interventions performed during the primary assessment focus on stabilizing the critical systems: respiratory, circulatory, and nervous systems. A critical step in the primary assessment is determining whether to continue the assessment on scene or begin transport and complete everything else en route to a hospital. Next, assess for specific injury or illness signs through a focused or rapid trauma assessment. Finally, evaluate the patient's medical history and perform reassessments.

- **Recognition of injury or illness**—As a result of the scene size-up and patient assessment, identify the illness or injury and the patient's priority for care and transport.
- **Patient management**—Employ appropriate care procedures, guided by protocols, with your patient's response to interventions and, at times, consult with medical direction to further guide your care. All patients need to be treated equally and with respect. Ongoing management is the paramedic's responsibility and begins immediately after making patient contact and continues until care is transferred at the emergency department.
- **Appropriate disposition**—Based on the results of your assessment, the effects of the care measures you have employed, and your system's protocols, you will determine the disposition of your patient. That disposition may bypass a local emergency department to go directly to a level I or II trauma center, a chest pain center, a designated stroke center, or a burn center. Some paramedic systems are beginning to institute a program whereby paramedics may determine to transport patients to urgent care or a physician's office instead of an emergency department. An additional possible disposition is to treat and release the patient with instructions to seek the advice of a personal physician.
- **Patient transfer**—The health care system is complex and facilities are often specialized; as a result, paramedics are often responsible for the safe and efficient transfer of patients from one facility to another. During this transfer, paramedics are not simply responsible for patient movement between facilities, but also ongoing patient care, including medication administration and reassessments.
- **Documentation**—At the conclusion of patient care, paramedics must document the results of their assessment and care to ensure the continuity of patient care. Documentation is objective and based on what was seen/observed and how patients responded to interventions.
- **Return to service**—At the end of a response, paramedics must ensure that they and their crew prepare the ambulance to return to service. This includes proper cleaning and refueling the vehicle, maintaining equipment, and replacing supplies used during the call.

3. **Give examples of additional responsibilities of paramedics.**   pp. 46–48

The responsibilities of paramedics extend beyond the emergency call and include:

- **Administration**—It is essential to identify strategies and complete tasks that help the system perform more efficiently. This includes checking expiration dates on drugs in the ambulances and store rooms, cleaning the stations, tracking waste, and maintaining positive working relationships with other agencies and the public.
- **Community involvement**—Paramedics promote and participate in programs to help the community recognize when EMS is needed, how to access the system, and how to provide basic life support (BLS) until the ambulance arrives. Community involvement also includes participation in the development and presentation of programs to improve health—stressing a healthy diet, for example—and to reduce injury, such as promoting seat-belt use or visiting the homes of elderly citizens and helping them identify and correct trip hazards. Maintaining regular community involvement improves the public's perception toward EMS and promotes a healthier community.
- **Support for primary care**—Modern health care is evolving in ways aimed at ensuring that costly resources are best directed to serve the patient most in need of those resources. In support of this aim, paramedics have an interest in providing injury and illness prevention to reduce unnecessary 911 activations and help the public understand when to visit their physician instead. Additionally, paramedics may transport or direct patients with minor injury or illness to alternative facilities such as urgent care centers or physicians' offices.
- **Citizen involvement in EMS**—Ordinary citizens can be highly important evaluators of the EMS system, because they are its consumers and can best say what elements of it are important to them. Pay attention to the comments, suggestions, and criticisms of patients/citizens you contact and pass what you learn along to the appropriate personnel in your system.
- **Personal and professional development**—To maintain and improve your ability to provide prehospital care, you must participate in professional development. This may include taking refresher and continuing education courses, engaging in skill maintenance exercises, and completing advanced courses to prepare for jobs in leadership positions or nontraditional work settings.

4. **Integrate expected characteristics of professionalism into all facets of
your practice of paramedicine.** p. 48

Professionalism refers to the conduct or qualities that characterize a practitioner in a particular field. Paramedics who maintain professionalism display evidence of self-regulation, meaning they hold themselves to high standards. These standards include their own personal ongoing education, daily work activities including vehicle and equipment checks, and in patient care. In paramedicine, paramedics recognize that they are providing a service to the community and seek out input from the community to identify how their job can be improved. After providing patient care, professional paramedics seek out how they can do better the next time and ensure their care meets accepted standards. Finally, paramedics promote continuously improving patient care by supporting ongoing quality assurance and improvement programs.

5. **Given a variety of EMS scenarios, identify and resolve ethical issues.** pp. 48–49

Ethics are the rules or standards that govern the conduct of a professional group. For paramedics, these ethics are identified in the 1978 NAEMT "Code of Ethics." It is important to understand these ethics because paramedics can regularly find themselves in challenging situations that may be influenced by their personal beliefs. For example:

- An African American paramedic found himself managing a 72-year-old Caucasian male complaining of chest pain. The patient made several racial slurs and the paramedic observed a Ku Klux Klan membership certificate hanging on the wall. However, because the "Code of Ethics" states ". . . *provides services based on human need, with respect for human dignity, unrestricted by consideration of nationality, race, creed, color, or status,*" the paramedic continued to explain to the patient that he is a professional there to provide care, performed a 12-lead EKG that identified a ST-segment myocardial infarction, and rapidly transported the patient to a chest pain center while initiating aspirin, nitroglycerine, oxygen, and morphine.
- Sarah was providing public relations services at a local skilled nursing facility to promote utilization of her ambulance service. While there, a nurse asked how Sarah's program's patient care compares to another ambulance's. Sara, following the "Code of Ethics," which states ". . . *groups of Emergency Medical Technicians, who advertise professional services, do so in conformity with dignity of the profession,*" stated that members of her service always strives to provide the best patient care they are able to and they perform regular continuing education and quality assurance for their members. She did not comment on the patient care provided by another service.

6. **Give examples of behaviors that demonstrate the expected professional
attitudes and attributes of paramedics.** pp. 49–52

The many attributes that professional paramedics demonstrate include:

- **Strong leadership**—Paramedics maintain a sense of calm on a stressful scene, communicate their needs clearly, and keep all personnel involved.
- **Integrity**—Paramedics acknowledge that we are all human and make mistakes. When a drug-math error occurs, the paramedic admits it, and tells the receiving hospital how much drug was actually given, charts the error, and makes no effort to hide the mistake.
- **Empathy**—After terminating a cardiac arrest in the field, paramedics clean up the room and the patient, making them presentable for the family to spend time alone with their loved one. They are attentive to the family's needs rather than rushing to go back into service.
- **Self-motivation**—Paramedics take the initiative, such as cleaning up a mess at the station as soon as they see it, even when it is not their own. They also seek out clarification on how to manage challenging patients in an effort to do better the next time they are faced with that situation.
- **Professional appearance and good hygiene**—Paramedics arrive at work ready for the day with a clean and ironed uniform, freshly showered, with (males) facial hair trimmed, and minimal jewelry. They keep a clean uniform in their personal vehicle or at work, so if their uniform becomes stained or soiled during a call, a clean one is available.
- **Self-confidence**—Be humble and accept limitations; when presented with challenging or unique situations, seek help from management, either from a supervisor or from medical control.

- **Good communication skills**—Paramedics spend time listening to the concerns of patients, families, customers, and the community. After listening to all of the pertinent information, the paramedic repeats it back to make sure he understands what was said.
- **Strong time management skills**—Some paramedics prefer changing into their uniforms at work. Those who do this arrive well before their shift begins so that they can change into their uniform before their shift starts. This way they are not caught by surprise when there is an emergency call waiting for them and as a result have a response delayed.
- **Teamwork**—Paramedics with strong teamwork skills recognize that everyone is trying to help the patient to the best of their ability. During stressful calls, particularly when things are not going well, team-oriented paramedics seek out the input of other team members, asking what ideas they may have, rather than trying to be the sole source of direction or ideas about patient care.
- **Respect for all others**—It is important to respect the beliefs of other religious and cultural groups. For example, if called to a mosque for an EMS call, be prepared to remove your boots prior to entering; although it may delay patient care a few minutes, it shows respect toward the religion's value systems and customs.
- **Patient advocacy**—Paramedics always stand up for their patients' needs. For example, when arriving at an emergency department, a nurse may want to place a paramedic's patient in a bed without a cardiac monitor. When paramedics know that the patient warrants continuous cardiac monitoring, they speak up for that need, and are willing to wait with the patient on the ambulance stretcher and cardiac monitor until the right bed is available—even if that means delaying going back into service, or getting out of work on time.
- **Careful delivery of service**—When paramedics recognize that they have not performed a high-risk and low-frequency skill for an extended period, they seek out a field training officer or a supervisor to review and practice the skill so that they maintain proficiency and can perform the skill when it is truly needed.

7. **Advocate for high standards of professionalism in EMS.** pp. 48–49

Paramedics can advocate for professionalism in a variety of ways. First and foremost is to promote high standards by example. On a peer-to-peer level, paramedics always follow the "Code of Ethics," and remind others of the code when they see behaviors that do not meet the code's ethical standards. They encourage participation in active quality assurance programs and professional organizations, and regularly attend continuing education programs. On a system level, paramedics promote high standards of professionalism by helping to identify ways to make the system work more efficiently, constantly working to maintain the public's positive impression of the program, and when they identify a problem, they proactively seek out a solution rather than waiting for someone else to fix the problem for them.

Case Study Review

Reread the case study on pages 40 and 41 in Paramedic Care: Introduction to Paramedicine; *then, read the following discussion.*

This case study demonstrates the coming together of personnel from many agencies to meet the prehospital needs of a patient—an EMS system.

The efficient response demonstrated by this call began well before the dispatch of Medic 49. Bobby Moore has maintained his certification throughout his career as a paramedic and is a master of assessment and prehospital emergency care. He checked his ambulance thoroughly that morning to ensure it was stocked with the necessary supplies and that all equipment was working well. He checked the oil, tire pressure, and fluid levels and tested all lights, sirens, and radios. He was ready to respond when the call came in.

Computers linked the incoming phone call reporting the emergency to a database that identified the location (an exact address) of the caller and any elements of medical history (such as the number of responses to the address, serious past medical history of patients at the address, or potential for violence at the address) linked to that phone number and address. This information was available on a computer in the ambulance as soon as the call was assigned and helped the paramedic better prepare for response and better ensure scene safety. A computer screen at the dispatch center displayed a map that highlighted the location of the caller and the closest police, ambulance, and fire units. Further enhanced computer-aided dispatch systems also highlight areas of likely traffic congestion, school zones, or road construction to help the dispatcher best direct the responding units to the scene.

Standardized prearrival instructions given by the emergency medical dispatcher helped the woman's husband regain his composure and take initial actions to protect his wife's airway and breathing. Without such steps, the stroke patient might have died or aspirated before EMS arrived. The conversation between the caller and the dispatcher may also help guide paramedics to the patient's side.

Bobby Moore viewed the scene and ensured it was safe, then moved quickly to his patient's side. There he provided assessment, care, and transport according to protocol, policies, and procedures. These established practices allowed Bobby to properly evaluate and recognize an acute stroke, determine its onset, and use that information to identify the appropriate destination hospital that could best treat his patient's condition. Bypassing the closest emergency department and transporting directly to a designated stroke center was a process set up ahead of time in his system's policies.

He demonstrated empathy and a sincere concern for his patient. He suspected that a stroke caused the patient's signs and symptoms and employed a quick stroke assessment scoring system that confirmed these suspicions. He knew a stroke is a time-sensitive emergency and limited his scene time by deferring his secondary assessment until he was in the ambulance and moving toward the proper hospital. As a result, the patient received quick therapy best able to help her.

Paramedic Moore's communication with the emergency department and the medical direction physician was effective—because he requested a "stoke alert," the physician immediately knew what Bobby was speaking about. This sped the response as the "stroke team" was awaiting the patient's arrival. As Bobby transferred patient responsibility to the physicians, he provided a quick update of the patient's condition and any changes in her signs and symptoms.

Because of the quick care provided by this EMS system and its paramedic, this patient experienced the best outcome possible with today's technologies. She was integrated into a system of primary care and can move quickly back into the mainstream of society.

Content Self-Evaluation

MULTIPLE CHOICE

_____ 1. The roles and responsibilities of today's paramedic are vastly different than they were 10 to 15 years ago.
  A. True
  B. False

_____ 2. Before responding to a call, you must be
  A. emotionally able to meet the demands of patient care.
  B. physically able to meet the demands of patient care.
  C. mentally able to meet the demands of patient care.
  D. sure the ambulance and equipment are ready for the response.
  E. all of the above.

_____ 3. Before responding to a call, you must be familiar with
  A. local EMS protocols.
  B. the local communications system.
  C. local geography.
  D. neighboring EMS agencies.
  E. all of the above.

_____ 4. A call involving which of the following is LEAST likely to require additional assistance?
  A. A single ill patient
  B. Reported use of a weapon
  C. Knowledge of previous violence
  D. Hazardous materials
  E. A rescue situation

_____ 5. Which of the following is an element of scene size-up?
  A. Identifying potential scene hazards
  B. Identifying the number of patients
  C. Determining the nature of the illness
  D. Requesting additional services
  E. All of the above

_____ 6. Which of the following is NOT an element of the primary assessment?
   A. Determining an initial patient impression
   B. Assessing patient responsiveness
   C. Ensuring the patient's breathing
   D. Investigating the patient's medical history
   E. Treating any life threats

_____ 7. The recognition of the severity of injury occurs during the
   A. scene size-up.   D. reassessment.
   B. primary assessment.   E. both A and B.
   C. physical exam.

_____ 8. An example of when a paramedic may elect to drive past the closest emergency department for a specialized hospital is when the patient is experiencing
   A. seizures.   D. dizziness.
   B. acute stroke.   E. shortness of breath.
   C. cardiac arrest.

_____ 9. You are responsible for patient care and therefore also ultimately responsible for selecting the transport destination for your patient.
   A. True
   B. False

_____ 10. When a patient receives a minor injury and is transported to an alternative care facility such as an outpatient clinic, this care is best described as
   A. basic care.   D. diversion of care.
   B. primary care.   E. health maintenance.
   C. treat and release.

_____ 11. Which of the following items is NOT an essential part of the transfer of a patient between health care facilities?
   A. A verbal patient report from the transferring primary care provider
   B. A copy of the essential parts of the patient's chart
   C. The results of all diagnostic tests
   D. A summary of the patient's past medical history
   E. A summary of the patient's present medical history

_____ 12. The patient-care report should normally be completed
   A. before arrival at the emergency department.   D. upon arrival at your base station.
   B. upon arrival at the emergency department.   E. either C or D.
   C. as soon as care is completed.

_____ 13. Why is it inappropriate for a paramedic to identify a patient as "being drunk"?
   A. It is an opinion.
   B. It is not an objective observation.
   C. It cannot be proven with the means available to the paramedic in the field.
   D. It subjects a paramedic to legal liability.
   E. All of the above are correct.

_____ 14. Which of the following is a component of returning to service after a call?
   A. Refueling the ambulance   D. Reviewing the call with the crew
   B. Restocking supplies   E. All of the above
   C. Stowing equipment

_____ 15. Which of the following is NOT a part of community involvement for the paramedic?
   A. Teaching CPR
   B. Transporting patients to alternative care facilities
   C. Conducting EMS demonstrations
   D. Providing prevention programs
   E. Sponsoring programs that help the public recognize when to access EMS

©2013 Pearson Education, Inc.
Paramedic Care: Principles & Practice, Vol. 1, 4th Ed.

16. What is the unique benefit of having citizen consumers involved in the development, evaluation, and regulation of the EMS system?
    A. They can help seek out alternative funding.
    B. They provide an outside, objective view of the EMS system.
    C. They do not have the prejudices of most EMS providers.
    D. They can provide insight into new care procedures.
    E. All of the above are correct.

17. As the volume of EMS responses increases, so should the hours of training for EMS personnel.
    A. True
    B. False

18. Participation in which of the following will help you maintain interest in EMS and maintain your skills and knowledge?
    A. In-hospital rotations
    B. Case reviews
    C. Research projects
    D. Mass-casualty drills
    E. All of the above

19. Ethics are laws that govern the conduct of members of a profession.
    A. True
    B. False

20. Which of the following is NOT an attribute of a professional?
    A. Leadership
    B. Excited demeanor
    C. Empathy
    D. Self-motivation
    E. Diplomacy

21. When presented with a complex situation, a self-confident paramedic will ask for assistance.
    A. True
    B. False

22. Which of the following is NOT a method of displaying empathy?
    A. Being supportive and reassuring
    B. Demonstrating respect for others
    C. Having a calm and helpful demeanor
    D. Accepting constructive feedback
    E. Understanding a patient's feelings

23. A paramedic shows respect for all patients by providing everyone with the best possible care regardless of their race, religion, creed, sexual orientation, or age.
    A. True
    B. False

24. Personal biases that are appropriate while you practice as a paramedic include which of the following?
    A. Religious
    B. Social
    C. Political
    D. Ethical
    E. None of the above

25. Placing the patient's needs above your own represents which professional attribute?
    A. Empathy
    B. Diplomacy
    C. Patient advocacy
    D. Initiative
    E. Self-confidence

MATCHING

Write the letter of the paramedic responsibility in the space provided next to the action to which it applies.

Responsibility

A. Preparation

B. Response

C. Scene size-up

D. Patient assessment

E. Recognition of illness or injury

F. Patient management

G. Appropriate disposition

H. Patient transfer

I. Documentation

J. Return to service

Action

_____ **26.** Refuel the vehicle.

_____ **27.** Follow patient-care protocols.

_____ **28.** Transport a patient to an outpatient center.

_____ **29.** Determine the mechanism of injury.

_____ **30.** Record the care you provided.

_____ **31.** Be familiar with local protocols.

_____ **32.** Determine the patient's medical history.

_____ **33.** Categorize the patient's priority for transport.

_____ **34.** Take a report from the sending facility.

_____ **35.** Drive responsibly and safely.

_____ **36.** Deliver a patient to a level II trauma center.

_____ **37.** Be mentally fit to respond to a call.

_____ **38.** Check crew members for signs of stress.

_____ **39.** Identify the nature of the illness.

_____ **40.** Determine the seriousness of the injury.

©2013 Pearson Education, Inc.
Paramedic Care: Principles & Practice, Vol. 1, 4th Ed.

4

Workforce Safety and Wellness

Review of Chapter Objectives

After reading this chapter, you should be able to:

1. **Define key terms introduced in this chapter.**

   Knowing and being able to apply the key terms in each chapter is critical to understanding chapter concepts. Write the list of key terms. Then write the definition of each one in your own words. Check your understanding by confirming the definitions in the text glossary. Correct any misunderstandings. Create a study aid by writing each key term on the front of an index card and the definition on the back. Use the cards to quiz yourself or to have someone quiz you.

2. **Given a variety of scenarios, recognize potential threats to safety and wellness.** pp. 57–58

   Because of the use of lights and sirens, the greatest threat to a paramedic's personal safety occurs during an emergent response. This is why the concept of exercising due regard is so important. Due regard means recognizing that different drivers will react differently to the approach of emergency vehicles. It also means that you must maintain an intense lookout for hazards while driving the emergency vehicle. You must anticipate the actions of other drivers on the highway, including those that are unexpected and not in keeping with the right of way given to you under the law. Otherwise you may find yourself responsible for injury, or injure yourself, when your intent was to provide care.

   Paramedics also pose a risk to themselves by lifting and moving improperly. Using the back to lift instead of the legs is an easy way to cause an injury that can cut short any career. It is important, especially in today's increasingly obese society, to ask for assistance lifting and always utilize safe lifting techniques. Many programs are now utilizing mechanized stretchers. These stretchers are designed to protect the back from lifting awkwardly. It is important to utilize these stretchers, whenever available. In addition to power stretchers, other devices have increased in availability to help reduce the potential for back injuries at key steps in the patient-care process. For example, slide boards are available to help slide a patient from a bed and onto the cot, and stair chairs are designed with tracks to help decrease back strain while moving patients down a set of stairs. Utilize these, and other injury prevention techniques, whenever possible to help reduce the chances of on-the-job injury.

3. **Explain the importance of preventing EMS workforce injuries and illnesses.**   p. 57

Work-related injuries and illness are an unfortunate and often preventable aspect of working in EMS. As an individual, experiencing a work-related injury/illness will not only cause days to weeks of lost working time (lost money), but it can also cut short one's career. For an organization, a serious work-related injury or illness can cause hundreds of thousands of dollars in workers' compensation, as a result of paying other providers overtime to cover open shifts, and due to disability payments.

Remember that even as a paramedic, work is just a job. There is no reason to sacrifice one's ability to enjoy life outside of work in an effort to help another individual. In an effort to reduce the potential for work-related injuries and illnesses, practice safe lifting techniques, always utilize safety equipment and clothing at accident scenes, wear appropriate body-substance isolation equipment, wash hands, and get adequate rest.

4. **Describe the role and elements of basic physical fitness in EMS workforce safety and wellness.**   pp. 57–58

Maintaining personal physical fitness has many benefits. It improves one's ability to perform the job; reduces blood pressure, heart rate, and stress; and increases metabolism, muscle mass, and the overall quality of life. In addition, increasing one's physical fitness decreases the chances of experiencing a work-related injury. This is particularly important, as significant portions of EMS providers are overweight.

There are three primary aspects to physical fitness: muscle strength, cardiovascular endurance, and flexibility. Increasing muscle mass is achieved through regular exercise targeted at training muscles to exert force and typically requires isotonic exercise. Cardiovascular endurance increases through regular intense exercise, at least three times per week, with an effort vigorous enough to increase the heart rate to a target level. This type of exercise can be achieved through active walking, bicycling, running, or swimming, for example. Finally, flexibility is just as important as cardiovascular endurance and muscle strength. Flexibility improves the range of motion for all joints and is best achieved through regular extended stretching by holding each stretch for at least 60 seconds.

5. **Explain the consequences of addictions and unhealthy habits.**   p. 60

The two most common EMS-related addictions are tobacco and caffeine. Smoking and the effects of nicotine are well known to be detrimental to respiratory and cardiovascular health and are linked to lung cancer. Smoking cessation programs using replacement therapy (nicotine patches), behavior modification, aversion therapy, hypnotism, and "cold turkey" approaches represent structured programs of controlled withdrawal from sociocultural, psychological, and physiological dependency on the drug. The result of a successful smoking cessation program is better respiratory and cardiovascular health and a reduced risk of respiratory infection and cancer. Caffeine addiction is exacerbated by poor sleep habits and excessive work hours. Work to minimize caffeine intake by assuring yourself of proper rest prior to shifts and limiting caffeine intake to the equivalent of two cups of coffee per day.

6. **Demonstrate work habits that minimize the risk of back injuries.**   pp. 60–62

Proper lifting and moving techniques, especially when coupled with good physical fitness and good nutrition, help protect the musculoskeletal system from the high risk for injury associated with prehospital emergency care. Good posture, lifting with the leg muscles, and keeping the back straight, the palms up, and the body close to the object being lifted will reduce the potential for injury. Exhale during a lift, keep your feet apart with one foot ahead of the other, take your time, and ask for help when you think you will need it. These principles will make lifting easier and help keep you from incurring back injury during your years of service.

7. **Given a variety of scenarios, select proper Standard Precautions for infection control.**   pp. 62–65

Standard Precautions (SP) practices include the use of personal protective equipment (PPE) to isolate the body from contaminants found in the air and body fluids while caring for a patient. These practices involve using protective latex or plastic gloves to protect yourself when touching a patient if there is reasonable expectation of contact with body fluids, including tears, vomit, saliva, blood, urine, fecal material, cerebrospinal fluid, or any other body fluid or substance. Masks and protective eyewear should be used whenever there is a reasonable expectation that fluid or droplets will be splattered, as is the case with arterial hemorrhage, endotracheal intubation, intensive airway care, childbirth, and the cleaning of contaminated equipment. When a patient has or is suspected of having tuberculosis or another highly contagious airborne disease, use of a special type of mask, either the high-efficiency particulate air (HEPA) or N-95 respirator, offers protection by removing small infectious particles from the air. Gowns are worn to protect clothing and the body from contamination by splashing of body fluids in extreme circumstances (like childbirth). A gown impervious to fluid movement is recommended. When possible, use disposable equipment for patient ventilation and other invasive procedures.

8. Discuss various patient, family, and EMS provider responses to death and dying. pp. 67–69

Even though paramedics are exposed to death and dying, they don't necessarily handle these events better than other people. All people tend to move through the same stages of the grieving process, although age and the patient's special circumstances may alter the presentation of those stages. The stages of the grieving process are: denial, anger, bargaining, depression, and acceptance. Everyone experiences these stages differently.

Children may not recognize the significance and finality of the event or may fear that death may soon happen to themselves or others. Adults react differently, usually experiencing a "paralyzing" feeling followed by intense grief for weeks. The intensity gradually subsides, with later peaks of feeling associated with anniversaries, birthdays, and the like. The elderly usually are concerned about the effects of the death on others and their loss of independence.

9. Respond professionally and compassionately to patients and family members in situations involving death and dying. p. 68

It is impossible to be completely prepared to deal with every death-related situation. When faced with a situation in which someone has died, the first step is to calm yourself and remind yourself that death is a natural process and it is OK to not be able to help the deceased individual. Before talking with the family, be sure to be free of anxiety, take a few deep breaths, and then calmly ask to talk with them. Place yourself at their level. If they prefer to stand, stand with them. Preferably though, ask to sit down with the family and position yourself to be at their eye level. Ask who present is the patient's closest relative and direct all comments to that person.

Begin by identifying yourself by first name and clearly identify your level of training. Clearly state you have evaluated their family member (the patient), and then continue by stating that they are deceased or dead. Using euphemisms such as "passed on" or "they are no longer with us" may seem more gentle; however, these euphemisms may create confusion and need to be avoided.

As appropriate for the situation, contact medical control, the police, or a medical examiner, and gain permission to remove any invasive equipment such as IVs or an endotracheal tube, so that the family may have time alone with the deceased. Clearly in some situations this cannot happen. Take a few minutes to prepare the patient for the family by covering the body, up to the shoulders, with a blanket, close the patient's mouth and eyes, and place a rolled up washcloth in the patient's hands. This last technique will position the deceased's hand in a cupping position that allows someone to hold his or her hand should a family member desire to do so.

10. Explain the pathophysiology of stress, including stressors, phases of the stress response, signs and symptoms, and consequences of prolonged exposure to stressors. pp. 69–71

The human stress response is the body's way of dealing with stress, and the outcome is either healthy or unhealthy. Healthy responses result in the individual's quickly adjusting to the stressor and physiologically and psychologically returning to normal. Unhealthy responses result in behavioral and physiological manifestations such as gastrointestinal disturbances, sleep disturbances, headaches, vision problems, fatigue, chest pains, confusion, a reduced attention span, poor concentration, disorientation, memory problems, inappropriate fear, panic, grief, depression, anxiety, and feelings of being overwhelmed, abandoned, or numb to emotion. A person with an unhealthy response may also experience withdrawal from normal social activities, increased use of drugs or alcohol, or inappropriate humor, silence, crying, suspiciousness, or activity levels.

Stress may become evident through almost any unusual behavior exhibited by the patient, family, or bystanders. It may manifest with hyperactivity or hypoactivity, withdrawal, suspiciousness, increased smoking, increased alcohol or drug intake, excessive humor or silence, crying spells, or any changes in behavior, communications, interactions with others, or eating habits. These behaviors can confound the assessment of the patient's mental status and place additional stress on the paramedic.

11. Describe effective stress management strategies. p. 71

Constructive mechanisms and management techniques used to deal with stress can be divided into two categories: immediate and long term. Immediate coping mechanisms include controlling breathing to reduce adrenaline levels and reduce heart rate, reframing thoughts to encourage or support any needed behavior on your behalf (e.g., saying to yourself "I can do this!"), and focusing your concentration on the responsibilities at hand (i.e., the needs of the patient), not the stressful problem. For long-term well-being, ensure your physical, mental, and emotional health. Exercise, watch your diet, and ensure supportive and pleasant distractions from the stress, such as a non-EMS circle of friends or a vacation away from the job.

12. Discuss the effects of shift work on the body and the ability to function effectively. p. 71

Emergency medical services providers always have, and always will, work shifts that allow for 24/7 operations. Inevitably, this causes some people to work outside of their normal circadian rhythm, which is the internal biological clock cycle. This internal cycle sets the intervals for several body functions, including appetite, temperature, sleep, and metabolism, to all slow down during a specific period—allowing the body to rest. Interrupting this cycle—for example, by working an EMS night shift—can stress the body's systems. This stress can lead to sleep deprivation, because the body is attempting to rest during peak shift needs and is running normally when we are trying to sleep before a night shift.

Although it is impossible to eliminate the need for night shift work, it is important to be aware of the risks associated with the shift. These risks include an increase in vehicle crash rates, increased medical errors, and increased chronic fatigue. These risks can be minimized by not working 24-hour shifts, identifying a set "anchor time" for daily guaranteed sleep (even when not working), sleeping in cool and dark environments, unwinding prior to sleep, and eliminating any stimuli that may interrupt the sleep cycle.

13. Describe the principles of psychological first aid. p. 73

Paramedics work in stressful environments and experience a significant amount of emotionally stressing events. In an industry that focuses on providing medical and emotional aid to the public, paramedics often forget to take some time to identify their own need for taking care of their own mental health. Following any significant single trying event, or whenever a paramedic feels the routine stresses of the job are beginning to wear, it is important to take the time to obtain some personal psychological first aid. Whether a witness, a friend, a fellow paramedic, or you need emotional help, the basic principles of psychological first aid are:

- **Contact and engagement**—Initiate contact with those in need of support.
- **Safety and comfort**—Provide a secure welcoming environment for dialogue.
- **Stabilization**—Remain calm and let the stressed individual relax.
- **Information gathering**—Identify what the stressed individual views as his or her needs.
- **Practical assistance**—Help to develop problem-solving strategies.
- **Connection with social supports**—Offer resources for a support system for problem solving.
- **Information on coping**—Suggest simple coping strategies that are proven to be successful.
- **Link to collaborative services**—Offer access to community support systems.

©2013 Pearson Education, Inc.
Paramedic Care: Principles & Practice, Vol. 1, 4th Ed.

14. Describe the role of disaster mental health services.   **p. 73**

The role of mental health services following a disaster is evolving. For years EMS providers and the public alike were offered critical incident stress debriefing (CISD); however, this practice has been shown to not only be ineffective, but it has actually been found to be harmful to the normal grieving process. Today, instead of a CISD, stress management that promotes emotional strength and decreases emotional vulnerability is being emphasized. This approach is proactive toward managing disaster events, rather than the reactive CISD format. The proactive approach to mental health care provides a more effective approach for dealing with emotional crises during a disaster.

Given this information, there is still a role for on-scene and intra-disaster mental health care. On-scene mental health providers can help identify victims and EMS providers experiencing abnormal stress-related symptoms.

15. Given a variety of scenarios, take steps to protect your personal safety, including effective interpersonal relationships and roadway safety precautions.   **pp. 73–74**

Maintaining personal safety is critically important. As EMS providers, paramedics are on the front line of the community, and are often viewed with great respect. Failing to return this respect to an individual creates a potential safety risk for the individual him- or herself and can also create safety risks for the next EMS providers that the offended individual interacts with. This can be avoided by treating everyone with dignity and respect; listening to their concerns, whether a patient or a witness; and acknowledging and honoring cultural differences and beliefs. Don't judge people because they believe or act differently; everyone is entitled to their own personal belief system.

As mentioned several times previously, responding to events and working on roadside incidents are the most dangerous situations EMS providers face. To help reduce the potential for personal harm, there are several practices worth following:

- Increase following distance, especially while responding with lights and sirens.
- Slow down when navigating intersections and corners.
- Always wear reflective safety vests while outside at roadway emergencies.
- Discourage the use of emergency escort vehicles.
- Assume no other vehicle sees the ambulance at an intersection.
- Maintain an awareness of adverse weather conditions.
- Find the safest parking location at any emergency.
- Always monitor for hazardous conditions.

Case Study Review

Reread the case study on page 56 in Paramedic Care: Introduction to Paramedicine; *then, read the following discussion.*

The case study presented identifies the evolution of Howard as a field paramedic. He came into the field with certain expectations, and after experiencing both physically and emotionally the consequences of not dealing with stress well, he has gained a healthy appreciation for his job and has learned the value of taking care of his own well-being. His short story, as presented here, serves as an example of how managing stress and taking care of your physical self improves both happiness and the ability to do the job of a paramedic.

After experiencing his own heart problems, Howard has taken an active role in maintaining his own physical health, which directly led to him being able to care for an injured patient. Howard admits he likely wouldn't have been able to do his job without his conscious decision to run and lift weights. Both of these activities increase cardiovascular endurance and body strength. He can now function longer under stress and is less likely to sustain serious injury because his body is strong and flexible. But that's not all that Howard has learned and taken to heart.

Howard displays a mature view of his actions to reduce his risks for injury and disease. He consciously employs Standard Precautions techniques and other safe practices to protect himself. He is aware that others are not as conscientious as he is, and he serves as a role model for others who are new to the profession. This attitude probably gains him the respect of his peers that he had tried to attain with his earlier "know-it-all" approach.

Howard has also gained an understanding of how stress affects both people in general and patients specifically. His personal experience of not managing stress well led to his limited "rebel" view and nobody wanting to work with him. Some personal re-evaluation and stress control helped him improve his ability to interact with people and patients during emergencies. His wake-up call changed him from a "cowboy" into the seasoned and caring paramedic he now is. It is this type of lifelong learning that is essential to your growth and maturation as a paramedic.

Content Self-Evaluation

MULTIPLE CHOICE

_____ 1. Most EMS injuries occur during lifting or while in or around motor vehicles.
   A. True
   B. False

_____ 2. All of the following are benefits of physical fitness EXCEPT
   A. decreased resting heart rate.
   B. decreased resting blood pressure.
   C. increased anxiety levels.
   D. enhanced quality of life.
   E. increased resistance to disease.

_____ 3. The core elements of physical fitness include all of the following EXCEPT
   A. disease resistance.
   B. muscular strength.
   C. flexibility.
   D. cardiovascular endurance.
   E. aerobic capacity.

_____ 4. Exercise performed against stable resistance, in which muscles are exercised in a motionless manner, is called
   A. isometric.
   B. polymeric.
   C. aerobic.
   D. isotonic.
   E. polytonic.

_____ 5. Improving cardiovascular endurance requires vigorous exercise at least ___ days per week.
   A. two
   B. three
   C. four
   D. five
   E. six

_____ 6. Flexibility is strengthened through
   A. isometric exercise.
   B. isotonic exercise.
   C. stretching.
   D. bouncing at the end of a range-of-motion exercise.
   E. weight lifting.

_____ 7. The most difficult challenge for EMS providers to overcome when trying to establish healthy eating habits is
   A. limiting carbohydrates.
   B. eating quickly.
   C. snacking between meals.
   D. overcoming bad habits.
   E. eating regular meals.

_____ 8. A proper and healthy diet minimizes intake of which of the following?
   A. Carbohydrates
   B. Vitamins
   C. Salt
   D. Protein
   E. Grains

©2013 Pearson Education, Inc.
Paramedic Care: Principles & Practice, Vol. 1, 4th Ed.

9. Water has what benefit over soft drinks?
   A. Cheaper
   B. More thirst quenching
   C. Better for you
   D. All of the above
   E. None of the above

10. Which of the following does NOT increase your risk for cancer?
    A. Prolonged, chronic, and unprotected sun exposure
    B. Consumption of charcoal-grilled foods
    C. Eating broccoli
    D. Being a postmenopausal woman
    E. Elevated cholesterol levels

11. Which of the following can reduce the risk of back injury?
    A. Doing abdominal crunches
    B. Quitting smoking
    C. Following good nutritional practices
    D. Getting adequate rest
    E. All of the above

12. Which of the following is NOT part of proper lifting?
    A. Positioning the load as close to the body as possible
    B. Locking your back in a slightly extended position
    C. Reaching while twisting to distribute weight
    D. Bending your knees
    E. Keeping your palms up

13. Because a person carrying a contagious disease may present without signs, you must consider the blood and body fluids of every patient you treat as infectious.
    A. True
    B. False

14. Which of the following infectious diseases is NOT transmitted via airborne pathogens?
    A. Hepatitis C
    B. Pertussis
    C. Tuberculosis
    D. Varicella
    E. Rubella

15. Which of the following items of personal protective equipment is/are recommended during oral suctioning of a patient?
    A. Gloves
    B. Eyewear and mask
    C. Gown
    D. Both A and B
    E. A, B, and C

16. Which of the following items of personal protective equipment is/are recommended when assisting a mother with childbirth?
    A. Gloves
    B. Eyewear and mask
    C. Gown
    D. Both A and B
    E. A, B, and C

17. HEPA and N-95 respirators are intended to protect against
    A. HIV/AIDS.
    B. tuberculosis.
    C. hepatitis B.
    D. hepatitis C.
    E. bacterial meningitis.

18. Proper hand washing requires
    A. removing rings.
    B. lathering hands vigorously.
    C. scrubbing vigorously for at least 15 seconds.
    D. scrubbing under fingernails and in creases of the knuckles.
    E. all of the above.

19. Which of the following is a recommended immunization for the paramedic?
    A. Tetanus/diphtheria
    B. Polio
    C. Hepatitis B
    D. Rubella
    E. All of the above

20. Used needles are to be disposed of by
    A. placing them in a properly labeled puncture-proof container.
    B. recapping them and placing them in a biohazard bag.
    C. returning them to the pharmacy for disposal.
    D. driving them deeply into the ground.
    E. breaking them and taping them together with the tips covered.

21. Sterilization uses which of the following to kill pathogens?
    A. Bleach
    B. Radiation
    C. EPA-approved chemical agents
    D. Pressurized steam
    E. All of the above except A

22. Which of the following represents the standard progression through the stages of grieving?
    A. Anger, denial, bargaining, acceptance, depression
    B. Denial, bargaining, anger, depression, acceptance
    C. Denial, anger, bargaining, depression, acceptance
    D. Anger, denial, bargaining, depression, acceptance
    E. Depression, anger, denial, bargaining, acceptance

23. A grieving patient who is withdrawing from friends and family and is unwilling to communicate with others is most likely in which stage of loss?
    A. Denial
    B. Anger
    C. Depression
    D. Bargaining
    E. Acceptance

24. Because paramedics experience death more often than the general population, they experience less stress and are better able to cope with it.
    A. True
    B. False

25. At which age are children most likely to feel that death is a temporary absence from which the deceased person will return?
    A. Newborn to age 3
    B. Ages 3 to 6
    C. Ages 6 to 9
    D. Ages 9 to 12
    E. Ages 12 to 18

26. When informed of the death of a loved one, some family members may explode in anger, throwing things and screaming.
    A. True
    B. False

27. When informing the family of the death of a member, use the words "dead" or "died" rather than less definitive ones such as "moved on" or "has gone to a better place."
    A. True
    B. False

28. The type of stress that has positive effects is
    A. distress.
    B. halcyon.
    C. stimulation.
    D. eustress.
    E. gravitas.

29. Which of the following is NOT a typical stressor for people working in emergency medical services?
    A. Shift work
    B. Violent people
    C. Waiting for calls
    D. Limited responsibilities
    E. Thirst

30. The human response to stress progresses through three stages, in this order
    A. resistance, alarm, exhaustion.
    B. alarm, resistance, exhaustion.
    C. alarm, exhaustion, resistance.

©2013 Pearson Education, Inc.
Paramedic Care: Principles & Practice, Vol. 1, 4th Ed.

D. resistance, exhaustion, alarm.

E. exhaustion, alarm, resistance.

_____ 31. The U.S. Surgeon General estimated that stress-related diseases kill approximately what percentage of people who die of nontraumatic causes?

A. 50 percent

B. 60 percent

C. 70 percent

D. 80 percent

E. 90 percent

_____ 32. The physiological phenomena that occur at approximately 24-hour intervals and regulate body temperature, sleepiness, and appetite are called

A. estrorhythms.

B. circadian rhythms.

C. lunar tidals.

D. fatigue/rest cycles.

E. solar epochs.

_____ 33. A recent study estimated that fatigue accounts for approximately how many motor vehicle crashes per year?

A. 5 percent

B. 10 percent

C. 20 percent

D. 30 percent

E. 35 percent

_____ 34. When you work a regular night shift, a technique that may help you maintain the appropriate awake/sleep cycle is

A. sleeping during one "anchor time" for both on- and off-duty days.

B. eating well before going to bed.

C. sleeping during the day after you work a night shift and at night when off duty.

D. sleeping in a warm place during the day.

E. taking short naps rather than long sleep.

_____ 35. Which of the following is a warning sign of stress?

A. Withdrawal

B. Feeling of being abandoned

C. Difficulty making decisions

D. Aching muscles and joints

E. All of the above

_____ 36. Which of the following is NOT a healthy behavior for dealing with or reducing stress?

A. Controlled breathing

B. Remaining distant from coworkers

C. Reframing

D. Establish non-EMS friends

E. Taking a vacation

_____ 37. Which of the following is a hazard commonly associated with auto crashes?

A. Downed power lines

B. Spilled hazardous chemicals

C. Moving traffic

D. Adverse weather conditions

E. All of the above

_____ 38. The best way to manage the mental health of paramedics is by offering support only following major incidents.

A. True

B. False

MATCHING

Standard Precautions

Write the letter or letters of the appropriate personal protective equipment necessary for each of the following procedures in the space provided.

A. Gloves

B. Mask and eyewear

C. HEPA or N-95 respirator

D. Gown

_____ **39.** Suctioning

_____ **40.** Childbirth

_____ **41.** Endotracheal intubation

_____ **42.** Patient with suspected TB

_____ **43.** Serious arterial blood loss

Special Project

Problem Solving

While transporting a patient to the hospital, you receive a needlestick from a used syringe that was left on the bench of your ambulance. List the steps you would take to reduce the chances of infection and complete the proper reporting process.

1. _____

_____

_____

2. _____

_____

_____

3. _____

_____

_____

4. _____

_____

_____

5. _____

_____

_____

©2013 Pearson Education, Inc.
Paramedic Care: Principles & Practice, Vol. 1, 4th Ed.

5 EMS Research

Review of Chapter Objectives

After reading this chapter, you should be able to:

1. **Define key terms introduced in this chapter.**

   Knowing and being able to apply the key terms in each chapter is critical to understanding chapter concepts. Write the list of key terms. Then write the definition of each one in your own words. Check your understanding by confirming the definitions in the text glossary. Correct any misunderstandings. Create a study aid by writing each key term on the front of an index card and the definition on the back. Use the cards to quiz yourself or to have someone quiz you.

2. **Explain the relationship between EMS research and EMS practice.**   p. 80

   When EMS first developed, there were few standards and no research to identify what interventions were beneficial and applicable for use in prehospital care. Thus, the practices implemented were drawn from other fields such as hospital and military medicine, and their use was based on conjecture and opinion.

   In today's EMS world, research has come to the forefront, and like most all other fields of medicine, research now drives the practices used in EMS today. Research looks at patient outcomes to determine if an intervention is beneficial, or even harmful. Through research, current practices are challenged, and potential new practices are explored. The goal of this ongoing research is to continuously improve patient survival and quality of life while decreasing morbidity. It makes no sense to continue practices that are ineffective at reaching these goals.

3. **Distinguish between the conclusions that can be drawn from research and those that can be drawn from more casual observations of phenomena.**   p. 80

   Ask a group of paramedics about the effectiveness of a given procedure, drug, or intervention, and every paramedic in that group will provide you with a subjective opinion based on their personal observations. Some of these paramedics will also tell you that their opinion is based on not only what they have seen, but also what their trusted colleagues have said. These opinions are anecdotal and have no means to be sustained other than through collective consensus. Research provides objective data to control outside influences on the intervention in question. By controlling for outside influences, the effect of the intervention being researched can be measured, and in the end clearly communicated. Thus, the conclusions obtained through controlled research are objective, and provide everyone with the same information on which opinions can be based. Such conclusions are not subjected to the bias of one's personal opinion and experiences.

4. Describe each of the steps of the scientific method. pp. 81–82

The scientific method strictly follows the following steps for research:

- *Observe and ask questions.* Identify something you're curious about and ask why, what, where, how, or when. Try to identify its process, causes, or consequences.
- *Conduct research, data collection, analysis, and synthesis.* Look up the topic of your question through scientific databases to determine what objective research has been performed and read the results. Reliable research sources for this information are available through academic institutions and research journals. A great source for this is PubMed.
- *Construct a hypothesis.* The hypothesis is the single statement a research project tests and either proves or disproves. A hypothesis is not a question, but rather the statement you hope to prove true or untrue. For example, a hypothesis may be "working a cardiac arrest on scene for at least 20 minutes improves overall cardiac arrest survival."
- *Test the hypothesis by experimentation.* Set up and perform a repeatable, objective experiment with clear parameters and controls. By scientific standards, experiments must be repeatable. In a true scientific experiment, only one variable may be tested/changed at a time.
- *Analyze results and draw conclusions.* Collect the results of the experiment and evaluate them. Typically, there must be a statistical analysis included to prove the hypothesis as true or untrue.
- *Revise the hypothesis.* In some situations, you may obtain the opposite result expected from the hypothesis being tested. In these instances, it is acceptable to revise the hypothesis. Changing the question allows the experiment to be run again, perhaps with slightly different variables or controls. Alternatively, when a hypothesis is untrue, it can be revised into the affirmative statement so that the research may be published with a proven hypothesis.
- *Report results.* After determining and evaluating the results, it is important to share them with others so that everyone can benefit from the information. Both expected and unexpected results are important to have published. Most medical research is published in peer-reviewed journals, which means that another researcher or field expert reviews the research paper prior to it being released in the journal.

5. Compare and contrast different types of research, including quantitative, qualitative, prospective, and retrospective approaches. pp. 82–83

Research can be described either with words or numbers. Quantitative research, which reports with numbers, is more common in medicine, because it is specific and objective. It compares a standard to a variable, and its analysis utilizes statistics. This research is good for looking at relationships, and in determining whether a hypothesis is true or untrue. Quantitative research is not as effective as qualitative research in determining why or how relationships exist. Qualitative research uses words and other non-numeric data to explain results. Quality assurance and customer satisfaction both rely more heavily on qualitative research than quantitative research.

Whether performing research qualitatively or quantitatively, it can be performed by either looking at existing data or by creating data during the experiment. Retrospective research looks backwards at existing data within a defined time period. This style of research is commonly used when looking for relationships or when evaluating existing practices. Prospective research requires an experiment to be designed first and then the hypothesis can be tested. When testing a new drug or intervention, it is essential to use prospective research. When comparing the benefits of retrospective and prospective research, retrospective studies can be done much faster because the results are already available. However, it is possible for retrospective data to be skewed or biased because potentially influential barriers cannot be controlled for.

6. Give examples of various experimental designs. p. 83

Designing the experiment is extremely important and requires consideration for the ethical treatment of the patients to be enrolled in the study. Ideally, all experiments would have patients randomly assigned into either the control or treatment groups in a double-blind manner. Double-blind means neither the patient nor the investigators know which group the patient is in during treatment. When this does happen, the research is considered an experimental study and the research is given the greatest amount of validity. Unfortunately, double-blind enrollment is not always possible. Often, complete randomization

©2013 Pearson Education, Inc.
Paramedic Care: Principles & Practice, Vol. 1, 4th Ed.

is not possible, or there is an ethical reason to control which patients are entered into either the control or treatment groups. When investigators maintain this sort of control, the research is considered quasiexperimental. Finally, observational studies do not have a control group. During observational studies, patients are all enrolled in some sort of treatment group. This often happens when there is a known and proven treatment that would be amoral to withhold—for example, if someone wanted to compare another drug to epinephrine for the treatment of severe anaphylaxis. No professional organization would consider withholding epinephrine ethically sound, and all patients in the study would need to receive epinephrine in some manner. Observational studies are common, but are considered less definitive than experimental studies.

7. **Describe different types of studies and their generalized levels of validity.** pp. 83–86

There are many different forms of studies. Most medical studies are performed in one of the following categories, which are listed in order from the greatest to the least validity:

- *Meta-analysis of randomized controlled trials.* A meta-analysis takes all of the data from a series of randomized controlled trials and combines it all together. Analysis is then performed on the data in aggregate to make conclusions.
- *Randomized controlled trials (RCT).* Randomized controlled trials are designed to randomly assign patients into the treatment or control groups. Although randomization can be achieved any number of ways, the study is generally either single or double blind. In single-blind studies the patients do not know which group they are entered into, and in double-blind studies, neither the patients nor the researchers know which group patients are in.
- *Nonrandomized controlled trials.* Nonrandomized controlled trials, which are quasiexperimental studies, allow researchers to assign patients into either the control or treatment groups. These studies are common when testing the benefits of new devices, such as a new laryngoscope blade to increase speed of intubation.
- *Cohort study.* Observational studies that compare a group of healthy individuals to a similarly sized group of patients who all have a given condition and are undergoing treatment over an extended period of time are called cohort studies. During the cohort study, the people within each group must be similar in some way. For example, an asthma drug may be studied in children, with one cohort being very urban patients and one cohort being rural patients.
- *Cross-sectional study.* Observational studies without a control group or without being carried out over the course of time are called cross-sectional studies. Cross-sectional studies look at a snapshot of time or are used for fixed single events, such as a leg fracture, heart attack, or current system barriers.
- *Case series.* A case series looks at a small group of patients, generally less than 50, with a similar condition. These reports are often used for identification of new conditions, such as when H1N1 was first recognized.
- *Case report.* When a structured critique or review of a single patient's care is presented, it is called a case report. Although not considered a research study, these can be beneficial for patients with unique presentations or disease considerations.
- *Expert opinion, editorials, and conjecture.* Groups of physicians, or single physicians, often document their collective professional opinions or beliefs about how patient care should be managed when there is no objective data available in a certain topic area. One example of this is when to determine that a hypothermic patient is dead. Because no patients will volunteer to be given severe hypothermia, and such a study would be unethical, there is only case reports of survivals that have been brought together to allow for expert opinions on the matter.
- *Animal research.* A significant amount of testing occurs on animals to see how certain chemical formulas, poisons, diseases, and so on affect organ systems and the biological process. This research is often performed when the medical community would consider carrying out such research on humans unethical.
- *Bench research.* Bench research is performed, literally, on a lab bench, and often in test tubes. It is important for learning, but is the baseline level of research. Although not often directly useful for medical practice, bench research is the foundation for other studies to be created and structured.

8. Given a published research article, discuss its validity. p. 86

Whenever an article is published, it is important to critique it in a manner where you ask if it is valid and applicable to your practice. Valid research is reproducible and has internal and external validity. For example, let's consider a critique of "Comparison of Perceived Pain with Different Immobilization Techniques," written by Drs. Cross and Baskerville and published in *Prehospital Emergency Care* (2001, 5:270–274). In this study, their hypothesis was that placing patients on a wooden spine board generates more back pain compared to a soft vacuum mattress. In looking for internal validity, we want to look for how the authors were able to rule out other causes of back pain. This is found in the methods, where they selected uninjured volunteers with no history of chronic or acute back problems. They also excluded anyone who had recently received any sort of analgesia. In looking for external validity, the study has to contain enough information to be reproducible and also be applicable to other patient groups.

The authors describe the wooden spine boards well, and describe the two different vacuum splint models used, which allows the study to be reproduced. However, in their own acknowledgement of study limitations, they state that the volunteer patients were comprised of a small group (18 people) of hospital employees. This allowed them an understanding of how to rate pain that the general population may not have. Just because the authors noted this limitation, which challenges external validity, the study is not invalid or valid. What it means is that yes, the study is applicable to other EMS providers, and yes the study can be reproduced, and yes the study showed the wooden boards increased back pain, but the level of back pain increase can be questioned because of the external factors mentioned.

9. Given a research proposal, identify the ethical considerations for human subjects that must be considered. p. 87

Research proposals that consider including human beings as the research subject must be evaluated for any potential ethical concerns. The ethical rules in use today are a combination of the Nuremburg Code of 1947, the Helsinki Declaration of 1964 (updated 1975, 1983, 1989, 2000, 2008), and the Belmont Report. These combined papers identify when patients must make an informed decision, that the research must respect human rights and dignity, and that the study must be aborted if there is evidence of actual harm to patients. Any academic institution performing research on humans must have an institutional review board that is charged with protecting human subjects and evaluating the ethical benefit and risks of the study.

10. Discuss the proper use of various descriptive and inferential statistics in a research study. pp. 88–89

Statistics can be used to either describe or make assumptions about a group of numbers, or a group that was studied. Descriptive statistics quite literally describe the data set and include the mean, median, mode, variance, and standard deviation. All of these numbers are intended to be presented together to demonstrate information about the data set and are used to describe the entire data set available. The mean is the average, and the median is the middle number. The mean is a good representation of normally distributed data sets, whereas the median better represents data sets with irregular data spreads. To determine how much change there is within the data set, or how large of a range the data set has, one must look at the variance and the standard deviation. The standard deviation is the square root of the variance, and the number most commonly reported to determine dispersion. The larger the standard deviation is, the more change there is within the data set.

On the other hand, inferential statistics make assumptions to larger populations based on the available data set. Because data sets usually represent a sampling of a larger population, inferential statistics are the assumptions made about the whole population based on the data set. Whenever reviewing inferential statistics, it is important to consider the sampling error, which is the assumed potential difference between the sampled data set and the entire population. The larger the sampling size, the more likely the sampling error is to be smaller, and the greater the confidence interval will be. The confidence interval is the measure of confidence that an inferred statistic is accurate. Most researchers aim for 95 percent confidence, and this is calculated based on a series of equations that consider the sample size, population size, and how many observations have been made. Essentially, inferential statistics suggest to us how the research applies to those outside of the data set.

©2013 Pearson Education, Inc.
Paramedic Care: Principles & Practice, Vol. 1, 4th Ed.

11. **Describe the purpose and intended content of each section of a research paper.** p. 90

When preparing a research paper, there are eight sections, listed next, that need to be written. Various sources allow for some blending of the discussion, limitations, and conclusion sections, but this would be handled specifically by any journal's guidelines. Each section is important, and must be accurate.

- The *abstract* begins every research article, and provides highlights of the research and conclusions. It is a short paragraph that summarizes the entire article, including why the research was performed, how it was performed, the results, and the conclusions, and is designed to tell readers why to read the entire article.
- Every article begins with an *introduction* that provides background as to why the research is needed, and includes all pertinent related research that has been completed. The introduction also provides the hypothesis that was tested.
- Because all research must be able to be repeated, the *methods* section must explain exactly how the research was carried out, how variables were controlled for, and how subjects were selected, and it must include a very specific description of what was done and how. This section must also include the names and models of any equipment used. Remember, this section provides the validity to the research and allows it to be repeated to be confirmed as true. To add to validity, the methods for all statistical analyses also need to be included.
- Immediately following the methods, *results* are presented. Often the shortest section of any research paper, the results section displays data in raw form on charts, tables, and graphs. If any results were excluded from analysis, they still need to be included in this section to prevent the assumption of bias.
- After sharing the results, the *discussion* section is where the data is interpreted and inferred statistics are applied to show how the new information discovered fits into and applies to the greater medical community.
- Within the discussion, and occasionally in a separate section, the *limitations* are identified. Limitations are any potential area that could allow for skewed data, research shortcomings, or areas that require further research.
- Finally, a *conclusion* explains whether the authors feel the hypothesis was proven or disproven by recapping the hypothesis and the primary findings.

12. **Describe how to perform a literature search.** p. 91

When preparing to perform a literature search, it is just as important to understand where not to go as it is to understand where to go. With the Internet providing so much readily available information, it is important to understand that most of the information out there is produced by individuals, and is not subject to peer reviews, the standard in medical literature. Thus, avoid websites, such as Wikipedia, that allow anyone to publish information on them. It is also generally a good idea to avoid .com websites and to try to stick to websites driven by academic institutions (.org) and ones that are directly affiliated with peer-reviewed journals. PubMed is a free Internet browser that permits access to nearly all scholarly peer-reviewed journals. It will provide free access to all abstracts and some journals. If you use PubMed from an academic institution, you will often have more journal access, as the school will have purchased access to many journals.

When reviewing literature for a research project, only consider previously peer-reviewed articles and articles that contain methods that can be reproduced. Generally, the more recent the research the better; however, landmark projects are those that drastically changed medicine or produced some new fundamental research and can be many decades old and still applicable.

13. **Given a variety of research papers, debate the merits of the study with your peers and instructors.** pp. 91–94

Review journals and choose two or three sample research papers. Answer the following questions:

- *Was the research peer reviewed?*
- *Was there a clear hypothesis or study purpose?*
- *Was the study type appropriate?*
- *What population were researchers studying?*

- *Were the control and study groups the proper size?*
- *Were the effects of confounding variables taken into account?*

14. Describe the role of published research reports in changing EMS practice.　　　　　　　　　　　　　　　　　　　　　　　　　　p. 94

Rarely does one paper fundamentally change medical practice significantly. Those papers that do are considered landmark papers. When a paper is published, it is important to consider it in the context of other related studies and also debate the impact of what the research means for the patients you serve, as well as the impact on the program. The more papers available that support a given practice, the stronger the evidence becomes to adopt that given practice.

As an example, for the last several years, research has been suggesting intubation is challenging and not consistently performed well by prehospital providers. This has led to the development of many non-visualized airway devices that can be rapidly deployed and utilized to deliver oxygen to patients, particularly those in cardiac arrest. At the 2012 National Association of EMS Physicians symposium, an abstract was presented that shows that one noninvasive airway, the King-LT airway, decreased cardiac arrest survival compared to intubated patients, and the research also showed that this was because the pressure exerted by the King's inflated cuff compressed the carotid arteries from the back of the oral pharynx and esophagus. Now, one could argue that this means that intubation needs to be performed: it is better. However, this needs to be placed in context with the skills of the providers on scene, the time it takes to intubate, the frequency of skill utilization, the quality of CPR, and the patients themselves. There may be a patient group that is better served with the King-LT that was not included in this study. This is just one example of how context is important, even when the research is outstanding.

15. Discuss the roles and responsibilities of EMS providers who participate in research studies.　　　　　　　　　　　　　　　　　　　pp. 94–95

For every research article published, someone initially asked a question. Asking a question is the first step in developing a research project. EMS providers have been, and continue to become, involved in research projects. When considering initiating or becoming involved in a research project, it is important to:

- Determine the question
- Prepare the hypothesis
- Decide what is being measured and how it will be measured
- Define the population being studied
- Identify study limitations
- Gain approval from proper authorities, including
  - Principal investigator
  - EMS directors
  - Any city/regional EMS agencies
  - State EMS agency (especially if a new drug or skill is being tested)
  - Medical director
  - Receiving hospitals in the study area (as applicable)
  - Internal Review Board (IRB) of hospital overseeing study
- Identify how patients will provide informed consent
- Gather data
- Analyze results
- Present data via
  - A conference
  - In a journal
- Follow up with more studies

©2013 Pearson Education, Inc.
Paramedic Care: Principles & Practice, Vol. 1, 4th Ed.

Case Study Review

Reread the case study on pages 79–80 in Paramedic Care: Introduction to Paramedicine; *then, read the following discussion.*

Although there is no patient in this case, this is a common conversation that has happened hundreds of times at ambulance services across the country.

Many paramedics, like Robert, began their careers similar to Steve. They knew of the "things we've always done." Few people questioned the time-tested practices. Robert has recognized though, that many of these "old" practices were performed because they seemed like a good idea—not because they were known to work. Originally, skills to perform and drugs to administer by paramedics were assigned because of tradition and opinion. Paramedics were told to perform these interventions and often were never given a clear explanation of why.

As Robert indicated he felt about MAST pants, there are many people who feel that skills that have been taken away from paramedics have worked. However, research is not just about expanding capabilities to new skills and drugs that work, but it is also about identifying interventions that may not work or may be harmful to the population as a whole.

Steve appears inquisitive, which is great. He is bringing up ideas that seem to work well on the surface, and likely these ideas were discussed in his classroom education. He wants to understand why they were "taken away." What he is learning here is that medicine is quite dynamic; it is constantly changing and evolving—this is why it is the *practice* of medicine. Steve is slowly realizing that today's interventions that we "know" work may one day be shown to also be ineffective and also go the way of the MAST pants. The drugs and interventions Robert discussed in this case were "known" to be the right thing to do when he was in school. It was likely shocking for him when each of them was taken away because of what research later demonstrated.

The important message from this case is that research is ongoing, and not every practice in place is based on research. Learn to ask "why" when being told to perform an intervention or administer a drug. Identify if it is a skill that is based on research or tradition. Be prepared for research to later challenge interventions that are currently based on tradition.

Content Self-Evaluation

MULTIPLE CHOICE

_____ 1. The primary goal of outcomes-based research is to improve
  A. morbidity.
  B. mortality.
  C. quality of life.
  D. patient care.
  E. all of the above.

_____ 2. Research is necessary to assure adequate reimbursement from insurance companies.
  A. True
  B. False

_____ 3. Which of the following is NOT a goal of EMS-related research?
  A. Eliminate ineffective skills
  B. Improve outcomes
  C. Expand the paramedic scope of practice
  D. Limit prehospital care
  E. Prevent further harm

_____ 4. The word *science* means
  A. knowledge.
  B. asking of questions.
  C. challenging the known.
  D. processed learning.
  E. objective truth.

5. The first step in the scientific method is to
   A. develop a hypothesis.
   B. identify what is already known.
   C. conduct research.
   D. review published research.
   E. ask a question.

6. "There is no difference in outcome between patients receiving full spinal immobilization and those receiving no spinal precautions during prehospital care." This is an example of a/an
   A. initial research question.
   B. study question.
   C. observation.
   D. null hypothesis.
   E. hypothesis.

7. It is acceptable to change the hypothesis during the scientific process.
   A. True
   B. False

8. Reporting research through a numerical representation of the data is
   A. qualitative research.
   B. quantitative research.
   C. mixed research.
   D. variable research.
   E. quasiexperimental research.

9. Which of the following research topics could be completed using qualitative research?
   A. Determining patient comfort following prehospital dislocation reduction
   B. Identifying the number of calls per shift completed before medication errors rise
   C. Identifying reasons why patients call 911 rather than seeking primary care
   D. Determining the cooling that occurs during 20 minutes of iced-saline administration
   E. Comparing intubation times between paramedics with and without OR experience

10. Retrospective research reviews existing data that is already available.
    A. True
    B. False

11. Prospective studies have a great opportunity for bias compared to retrospective studies.
    A. True
    B. False

12. Patients not receiving the treatment or drug being researched are placed in which group?
    A. Treatment
    B. Experimental
    C. Observational
    D. Baseline
    E. Control

13. What type of study does NOT have a patient group that has treatment withheld?
    A. Prospective
    B. Experimental
    C. Observational
    D. Randomized controlled
    E. Quasiexperimental

14. The study type that is given the greatest weight for validity is the
    A. meta-analysis RCT.
    B. randomized controlled trial.
    C. cohort study.
    D. case series.
    E. case report.

15. In a case series, neither the patient nor the physician knew during the research whether the patient did or did not actually receive treatment.
    A. True
    B. False

16. Research performed *in vivo* is
    A. bench research.
    B. animal research.
    C. a case report.
    D. a cohort study.
    E. retrospective.

17. External validity exists when research results can be applied to populations in other areas and regions.
   A. True
   B. False

18. The founding set of guidelines dictating the ethical treatment of humans during research was produced in the
   A. Napoleon Code.   D. Helsinki Declaration.
   B. Nuremburg Code.   E. Belmont Report.
   C. Bible.

19. A committee that reviews, monitors, and approves human research is called a/an:
   A. research quality committee.   D. institutional review board.
   B. medical monitoring committee.   E. independent review board.
   C. safety and survival committee.

20. Which of the following is a descriptive statistic?
   A. Mean   D. Standard deviation
   B. Median   E. All of the above
   C. Mode

21. Considering the following data set, determine the mean.

   | 24 | 34 | 34 | 53 | 34 | 23 | 63 | 98 | 31 | 53 | 67 |
   | 87 | 50 | 49 | 09 | 97 | 23 | 33 | 38 | 21 | 75 | 28 |

   A. 34   D. 36
   B. 46.5   E. 22
   C. 25.3

22. Considering the following data set, determine the standard deviation.

   | 24 | 34 | 34 | 53 | 34 | 23 | 63 | 98 | 31 | 53 | 67 |
   | 87 | 50 | 49 | 09 | 97 | 23 | 33 | 38 | 21 | 75 | 28 |

   A. 34   D. 36
   B. 46.5   E. 22
   C. 25.3

23. The section of a research paper that identifies study limitations is the
   A. abstract.
   B. methods.
   C. results.
   D. discussion.
   E. summary.

24. An article's abstract is likely to discuss the
   A. hypothesis.   D. conclusion.
   B. research methods.   E. all of the above.
   C. results.

25. When using the Internet to explore the literature surrounding a potential research topic, the most reliable search tool is
   A. bing.com.   D. PubMed.
   B. wikipedia.com.   E. google.com.
   C. research.org.

26. Most human-based research studies will not be accepted by the medical community if the research did not have
   A. IRB approval.
   B. peer review.
   C. a control group.
   D. double-blinded research.
   E. a null hypothesis.

27. Confounding variables are those that
    A. produce false positives.
    B. require additional research.
    C. increase study validity.
    D. may affect study outcomes.
    E. require different control groups.

28. It is important to identify what statistical analyses will be performed on results prior to obtaining the data to avoid
    A. bias.
    B. confounding variables.
    C. data dredging.
    D. low p-values.
    E. false negatives.

29. The principal investigator is the individual who
    A. asks the initial question.
    B. develops the hypothesis.
    C. oversees the entire study.
    D. collects all of the data.
    E. must have a PhD or MD.

30. Multiple randomized controlled trials that have had a meta-analysis performed are the most likely reports to generate what level of certainty/evidence?
    A. Level A
    B. Level B
    C. Class I
    D. Class II
    E. Class III

31. Delaying defibrillation or ventricular fibrillation for a patient in order to perform endotracheal intubation would be an example of a treatment with what recommendation?
    A. Level A
    B. Level B
    C. Class I
    D. Class II
    E. Class III

Special Project

Find any article online that discusses the benefits of adding a second medical helicopter to a transport region and its effect on patient mortality, and then critique the article by answering the following questions.

A. What was the hypothesis? Was there a null hypothesis?

_____

_____

_____

_____

_____

_____

_____

B. What was the experimental design? How does this affect validity?

_____

_____

_____

_____

_____

C. How does this study affect patient care in your area?

_____

_____

_____

_____

_____

_____

_____

D. Can the results be attributed to any other factors? What do you feel could have skewed the results?

_____

_____

_____

_____

_____

_____

_____

6 Public Health

Review of Chapter Objectives

After reading this chapter, you should be able to:

1. **Define key terms introduced in this chapter.**

   Knowing and being able to apply the key terms in each chapter is critical to understanding chapter concepts. Write the list of key terms. Then write the definition of each one in your own words. Check your understanding by confirming the definitions in the text glossary. Correct any misunderstandings. Create a study aid by writing each key term on the front of an index card and the definition on the back. Use the cards to quiz yourself or to have someone quiz you.

2. **Identify EMS roles that are within the domain of public health.**   pp. 103–105

   The overarching goal of public health is to rapidly identify potential hazards, identify emerging diseases and illness, and prevent disease outbreaks and injuries from occurring by taking as many steps as possible to identify and control risks. EMS providers are in a unique position to promote this process, because they have a finger on the pulse of the public health system. By working together as a system, EMS providers must:

   - Recognize and report developing disease clusters, suspicious activities, and injury clusters. For example, there may a sudden spike in similar illnesses following the opening of a new factory.
   - Identify areas and situations presenting high risk for injury.
   - Provide individuals and families access to resources to improve home health and safety.
   - Promote public health by taking the time to educate patients and families during situations of patient-care refusals.
   - Visit high-risk groups such as the elderly and impoverished youth and provide them information about proper health.
   - Aid in disaster management beyond recovery. In the weeks and months following a disaster, EMS providers have a key role in helping restore health and safety to affected communities.
   - Aid in data collection by tracking, through computer-aided software, changes in call and emergency request demographics.
   - Be empowered to act on observations made. No public health plan will work without the support of and follow-through from leadership within different organizations.

3. **Describe the components that must be in place for EMS and public health to work together.**   p. 100

   In order for EMS integration into public health to succeed, there are many components that must be working together to ensure that the entire public health system is set up for success. Both EMS and public health medical directors must coordinate efforts together to share goals and have a common vision for the outcomes of different projects. Further, there must be a collective desire to ensure EMS providers and other public health workers are educated as to each other's capabilities, limitations, and intended role in public health. Everyone must work together through regular meetings, planning, team building, and constant communication to build and maintain strong relationships between the leaders of involved organizations. Community involvement in the planning of coordinated public health initiatives is also essential. Disaster plans developed through public health initiatives must be locally planned and coordinated, practiced, and shared with the public. Finally, adequate funding must be available for these shared public health projects.

4. Discuss ways in which public health efforts have improved the quality of life.
p. 101

Public health initiatives have already made significant impacts in injury and illness prevention. The average individual's quality of life has been improved and enhanced, and the life span has been made safer and longer, directly and indirectly from many projects that have been completed, including:

- Pediatric vaccination standards and requirements
- Motor vehicle construction rules, speed laws, and safety requirements
- Introduction of workplace safety standards, including use of helmets, safety goggles, chemical handling, protection from extreme heat/cold, shift length, and pay
- Preventative management for coronary artery disease and stroke, including education on the importance of taking aspirin as soon as symptoms are suspected
- Hand-washing regulations for public and food-related workers
- Food safety through safe food handling, temperature controls, and animal handling
- Limiting exposure to second-hand smoke
- Family planning and access to prenatal care for impoverished families
- Nutrition-driven school food programs

5. Recognize the three categories of public health laws.
p. 101

Public health laws are divided into three categories based on their intended purpose:
1. *Illness and prevention*
2. *Police powers for public health agencies*
3. *Epidemiological tools*

6. Explain the basic concepts of epidemiology.
pp. 101–102

The branch of medicine that works to detect the sources of infectious disease epidemics and addresses the incidence and prevalence of diseases in large populations is *epidemiology*. Although this is a very large and multifaceted field, there are many constant concepts employed by epidemiology, such as the following:

- **Years of productive life**—Determined by subtracting the age at death from 65 (the normal retirement age). This may be increased to 70 in the next few years as society's average age increases.
- **Injury**—Damage to an individual as a result of acute exposure to external energy forces or the deprivation of essential needs such as heat, water, or oxygen. Injuries may be unintentional or intentional.
- **Injury risk**—The chance of sustaining injury from a hazardous or potentially hazardous situation.
- **Injury surveillance program**—The continuous reviewing and sharing of the analytic interpretation of continuously and systematically collected injury data. An injury surveillance program is essential for the continuous safety of public health individuals, and for effective planning and implementation of public health plans.
- **Preliminary prevention**—Strategies implemented to keep injury from ever occurring and to keep individuals from being exposed to a specific disease or illness. For example, many childhood immunizations are preliminary prevention strategies.
- **Secondary prevention**—The immediate medical care and management of an injury or illness that has occurred with the intent of stoppings its progression to minimize the symptoms or signs that develop.
- **Tertiary prevention**—The rehabilitation following an injury or illness to return an individual to full health.

©2013 Pearson Education, Inc.
Paramedic Care: Principles & Practice, Vol. 1, 4th Ed.

7. **Give examples of how EMS providers can be involved in injury prevention.** p. 103

Paramedics can intervene at the scene of an illness or injury and take advantage of a teachable moment. In a nonjudgmental, nonthreatening way, paramedics may identify behaviors that would prevent illness or injury—for example, wearing protective equipment such as seat belts in a car or helmets when biking—and instruct the patient as well as any witnesses in their use. Paramedics may also identify community risks such as improperly enclosed swimming pools, which are common sites of child drownings, or poorly protected railway crossings, which are likely sites of train-versus-auto collisions. When these community-wide risks are identified, it is important for paramedics not to just note them, but follow established communication pathways to make sure such risks are reported and followed up on. Without good communications between departments involved in public health, such a report would likely make it to EMS leadership and then become halted. Proactively knowing the players in different organizations promotes the speed at which risks can be mitigated.

8. **Describe the roles of EMS organizations and EMS providers in the prevention of EMS provider illness and injury.** pp. 105–106

Many individuals in the public look up to EMS providers; the actions of EMS organizations and crew members speak loudly. Citizens are less likely to listen to suggestions for improvement made by individuals who are not looking out for their own personal safety and well-being as well. Additionally, it does no EMS provider any good to become ill or injured during the course of their work: doing so takes away an experienced public health professional and also costs both the EMS organization and provider money.

Promote personal and partner well-being and safety by following a few commonsense but quite important practices. Always utilize Standard Precautions. This includes wearing gloves on all calls, and masks, gowns, and goggles when appropriate. Take time out of each day to get regular exercise. Exercise improves physical and immune system strength. In addition to regular exercise, eat well. Proper diet promotes healthy body functions and boosts the strength of the body's systems. To reduce the risk of back injuries, always utilize safe lifting techniques. Never twist or reach while lifting, use the legs and knees for lifting rather than the back, and never hesitate to ask a few extra people to help lift a heavy patient or object.

Maintaining emotional health is just as important as maintaining physical health. To maintain emotional health, maintain a work-life balance, have regular stress management strategies, keep side jobs unrelated to EMS, and take regular vacations. When emotional stress rises, and standard relaxation techniques do not work, seek professional health early. Most EMS organizations offer access to professional counseling as a job benefit. Take advantage of these resources, as the constant stress of major disease, trauma, tragedy, and upset patients does wear on everyone over time.

Safety at work can never be compromised. A safe mentality must begin prior to beginning a shift. During a shift, pay particular attention to safety during periods of increased injury risk. These time periods include emergency vehicle operations and while on the scene of any emergency. Emergency vehicle operations include the time spent as a driver and as a passenger. When driving, always maintain safe speeds, obey traffic warning signals, utilize due regard, and be mindful of factors that change hazards, including traffic density, uncontrolled intersections, other individuals, and the weather. As a passenger, whether in the front or back of an ambulance, always wear a safety belt, secure loose objects, and avoid distracting the driver. While on scenes, be mindful of all potential and actual risks. One recent risk mitigation strategy that stemmed from public health initiatives was a federal law requiring ambulances to be painted with highly reflective paint schemes on the rear of vehicles and the use of reflective vests by all personnel on the scene of highway emergencies.

9. **Identify areas of need for prevention programs in the community.** pp. 107–108

In reality, there are endless areas where communities can benefit from injury and illness prevention programs. Part of a healthy public health program is the identification of those areas at highest risk and prioritizing programs to do the greatest good for the greatest amount of people.

Infants and children have many public health needs for both injury and illness prevention. Infants have weakened immune systems compared to adults. For the first several years of life, children are unable to recognize and remove themselves from situations that increase their risk for illness, such as life in an unsanitary situation, being surrounded by second-hand smoke, and spending time near ill individuals. Additionally, because one of every three deaths for those under age 18 is injury related, it is important to help raise injury risk awareness and provide prevention strategies. For example, many children's trauma centers regularly teach bicycle safety and give away bike helmets in an effort to help decrease head-injury rates. Another example of a prevention strategy is car-seat safety checks offered by many fire departments and EMS organizations.

Motor vehicle collisions remain a leading injury-related cause of death in the United States, and alcohol is often a factor. Despite many regional and national programs to decrease drunken driving rates and improve safety belt use, it is important to continuously develop additional safe-driving technique and strategy programs.

As people age, their risks for injuries following falls and the number of medications they take both increase. EMS organizations can help mitigate fall risks by visiting the homes of elderly, helping them identify at-home fall and other risks, and employing strategies to reduce these risks. For example, remove small throw rugs, help install rails in the bathrooms, and turn down the temperature from water heaters (decreases burn risks). Elderly patients on multiple medications have two associated risks. First, they have an increased potential for accidentally overdosing on a medication should they forget which medicine they took and when. Additionally, especially when money is tight, many elderly individuals elect to skip medicine doses, or only take half doses, in an effort to make medicines last longer—even though this increases their health problems. These drug risks can be mitigated through education, helping individuals sort medicines, and providing access to drug discounts.

Finally, despite many good intentions, workplace injuries remain common. It may make sense for some EMS organizations to offer to travel to various work sites and provide feedback at the risks they observe and offer solutions to improve prevention and decrease some risks.

Case Study Review

Reread the case study on pages 99–100 in Paramedic Care: Introduction to Paramedicine; *then, read the following discussion.*

This case study visits an incident that highlights the consequences of not having an injury and illness prevention program in the community and provides an opportunity to examine the impact such an incident might have on EMS providers.

It is a hot July day and the fun-loving antics of a couple of children have turned into disaster. And what appears to be an accident was truly a predictable and preventable incident. This incident also demonstrates the discouraging results of some EMS responses and the stress they may cause those who provide care.

How would this scenario have turned out if John's parents had insisted that the pool be fenced in when it was installed to prevent the children from entering unsupervised? What if John and Timmy had attended a water safety and swimming course when the pool was installed? Would the outcome have changed if the EMS system provided caller instructions and John's mom had performed mouth-to-mouth ventilations on Timmy for the 6 minutes before the ambulance arrived or, better yet, if she had completed a CPR course and provided rescue breathing and chest compressions? As you can see, there were many opportunities to improve the chances for a better outcome from this incident through illness and injury prevention.

This incident also presents what must have been a very discouraging call for the care providers. Initially the paramedics must have felt good about their actions. Timmy showed signs of responding to treatment and hopes were high. However, as time passed, they became aware that their resuscitation was fruitless, leading to a costly and emotional burden on Timmy's parents as well as John and his parents. If the paramedics have children, they may be especially affected by the incident's result. If these providers, and the system they respond in, do not recognize this and deal with this stress, it may lead to job dissatisfaction and, eventually, to the paramedics leaving the profession.

As the EMS system matures, its members must become more responsible and active in identifying risks to the community and suggesting, supporting, and possibly sponsoring prevention education programs. We must also appreciate the impact critical incidents have on us as providers and be ready to request and accept assistance when they affect us.

©2013 Pearson Education, Inc.
Paramedic Care: Principles & Practice, Vol. 1, 4th Ed.

Content Self-Evaluation

MULTIPLE CHOICE

_____ 1. Which of the following has NOT been a public health accomplishment in the United States?
   A. Increasing vaccinations
   B. Increasing workplace safety
   C. Decline in infectious disease rates
   D. Increased water safety
   E. Decreased abortion rates

_____ 2. Public health is defined as the science and practice of protecting and improving the health of a community through the use of preventive medicine, health education, control of communicable disease, application of sanitary measures, and monitoring of environmental hazards.
   A. True
   B. False

_____ 3. The calculation made by subtracting a person's age at death from 65 produces a result called the
   A. years of productive life.
   B. injury risk factor.
   C. secondary span.
   D. epidemiological age.
   E. vital factor.

_____ 4. For effective EMS integration into the public health plan, which of the following must be in place?
   A. Strong medical oversight for both EMS and public health
   B. Aggressive pursuit and securing of funding
   C. A desire for emergency care workers and other public health providers to understand each other's roles
   D. Community stakeholder involvement in the planning process
   E. All of the above

_____ 5. A systematic method to collect, analyze, and interpret information about injury data is a/an
   A. injury risk program.
   B. injury surveillance program.
   C. epidemiological intervention.
   D. secondary prevention program.
   E. risk data analysis.

_____ 6. EMS providers' recognition of several patients developing the same illness-like symptoms and reporting their findings to officials would fall under the EMS responsibility of
   A. health promotion.
   B. disease surveillance.
   C. disaster management.
   D. injury prevention.
   E. fund raising.

_____ 7. EMS providers are well distributed throughout the population, are often considered to be champions of the health care consumer, and are high-profile health care role models.
   A. True
   B. False

_____ 8. A personal wellness program should include all of the following EXCEPT
   A. regular psychological counseling.
   B. a proper diet.
   C. strength training.
   D. cardiovascular fitness.
   E. a health-minded attitude.

_____ 9. Which of the following is essential to safe emergency driving?
   A. Being familiar with and obeying the traffic laws
   B. Understanding the capabilities and limitations of your vehicle
   C. Being able to handle weather and road conditions with precision
   D. Using proper sound and visual warning devices
   E. All of the above

_____ 10. A paramedic should enter a hazardous scene only when the proper rescue, utility, or hazardous materials teams are not available.
A. True
B. False

_____ 11. Which of the following statements about premature and low-birth-weight infants is NOT true?
A. There are close to 300,000 of these infants born each year.
B. These infants are far less likely to die in the first year of life.
C. More than 4,000 of these infants die each year.
D. Some of these infants have serious disabilities such as mental retardation.
E. Inadequate prenatal care is often a major factor in these births.

_____ 12. What percentage of child deaths is the result of injuries?
A. One-third
B. One-quarter
C. One-fifth
D. One-sixth
E. One-tenth

_____ 13. Which category of public health laws is considered the most controversial?
A. Illness and prevention
B. Mandatory vaccinations
C. Police powers for public health agencies.
D. Public safety enforcement
E. Epidemiological tools

_____ 14. Distributing child bicycle helmets and teaching proper fitting during a health fair is an example of
A. health promotion.
B. disease surveillance.
C. disaster management.
D. injury prevention.
E. fund raising.

_____ 15. Alcohol is a factor in over half of all fatalities related to motor vehicle crashes.
A. True
B. False

_____ 16. The greatest cause of preventable injuries in the geriatric population is
A. skeletal failure.
B. motor vehicle collisions.
C. falls.
D. intentional mechanisms.
E. burns.

_____ 17. The early release of patients from health care facilities to help control health care costs is likely to cause an increase in the number of EMS responses.
A. True
B. False

_____ 18. Which of the following is an action you should take as an EMS responder to implement injury prevention strategies?
A. Preserve response team safety
B. Recognize scene hazards
C. Engage in on-scene education
D. Know your community resources
E. All of the above

Special Project

Look up federal and local public health laws and regulations, and then categorize them into each of the three public health law categories below. Find at least three laws for each category.

A. Illness and prevention

_____

_____

©2013 Pearson Education, Inc.
Paramedic Care: Principles & Practice, Vol. 1, 4th Ed.

_____

_____

B. Police powers for public health agencies

_____

_____

_____

_____

C. Epidemiological tools

_____

_____

_____

_____

7

Medical/Legal Aspects of Prehospital Care

Review of Chapter Objectives

After reading this chapter, you should be able to:

1. Define key terms introduced in this chapter.

Knowing and being able to apply the key terms in each chapter is critical to understanding chapter concepts. Write the list of key terms. Then write the definition of each one in your own words. Check your understanding by confirming the definitions in the text glossary. Correct any misunderstandings. Create a study aid by writing each key term on the front of an index card and the definition on the back. Use the cards to quiz yourself or to have someone quiz you.

2. Describe the legal, ethical, and moral obligations of the paramedic.   **pp. 114–115**

A paramedic's legal responsibility to the patient and others is defined by statute, regulation, and common law. Failure to meet this responsibility may result in criminal or civil liability. Ethical responsibilities are those actions expected of a paramedic by the health care profession and by the public. Moral responsibilities are personal values of right and wrong and are governed by conscience. Legal, ethical, and moral factors guide an individual in his actions as a paramedic.

3. Describe the four primary sources of law.   **p. 115**

There are four primary sources of law in the United States: constitutional, common, legislative, and administrative. Constitutional law defines governmental authority and gives the individual certain rights. Common law is based on past judge-decided cases (case law) and is a fundamental principle of our legal system. Legislative law consists of statutes enacted at the federal, state, or local level. Administrative law consists of the regulations and rules that a governmental agency uses to implement legislative law. These four sources of law affect the legal responsibilities of the practicing paramedic.

    Civil law is noncriminal legal action between individuals for such things as matrimonial, contract, and personal injury disputes. It may also include civil wrongs such as assault, battery, medical malpractice, and negligence. Criminal law addresses actions against society (crimes) such as rape, murder, and burglary and will fine or imprison those found guilty.

4. Differentiate between civil and criminal law.   p. 115

Regardless of a law's source, each law passed is categorized as either a criminal or a civil law. Laws categorized as criminal laws are enforced by a federal, state, or local governing body. This governing body also prosecutes individuals violating these laws on behalf of society. Individuals who are convicted of violating criminal laws are subject to imprisonment, fines, or both. Civil laws, on the other hand, generally require an individual or organization to initiate a lawsuit against one or more defending parties. These are noncriminal cases and may include: personal injury, marital disputes, libel or slander, and contract violations.

5. Explain the concept of tort law as it applies to paramedic practice.   p. 115

A special branch of civil law, *tort law*, involves civil wrongdoings committed by one individual against another. These laws are particularly important to paramedics because tort law includes negligence, medical malpractice, and assault and battery. Should a patient or family ever claim a paramedic failed to provide adequate patient care, or that a paramedic's care caused the patient harm, any lawsuits would be filed under tort laws.

6. Outline the events that occur in a civil court.   pp. 115–116

In today's society, becoming involved in a civil lawsuit is unfortunately common. Paramedics can become involved in civil lawsuits for a variety of reasons, ranging from personal gross negligence to lawsuits involving accidents they responded to. In the majority of cases when paramedics are involved in lawsuits, it is likely because the paramedic happened to provide care for someone injured and the given paramedic just happened to be the one providing care. Because becoming subpoenaed for a lawsuit can be stressful for anyone, it is important to understand the events that occur during a civil lawsuit process. The events of a lawsuit include:

- *Incident.* The unintentional or intentional event that affected an individual or group.
- *Investigation.* An attorney's initial fact-collecting inquiry to establish merit for the case.
- *Filing of the complaint.* The plaintiff's formal petitioning of a complaint to the court. This petition must establish a legal basis for the claim, note the specific allegation of wrongdoing, and identify the parties involved.
- *Answering the complaint.* The official filling of the defendant's answer to each allegation with the court system.
- *Discovery.* The pretrial fact-finding mission completed by both sides of the case during which all relevant information is shared with both sides; includes examinations, interrogations, and document reviews (e.g., EMS reports). Often, this is the longest phase of any case.
- *Trial.* The formal presentation of the facts by each side of the case in a courtroom before a judge and in some instances a jury.
- *Decision.* The fair evaluation of the facts by the judge or jury to determine the defendant's liability and what, if any, damages should be awarded.
- *Appeal.* The request by the losing party for an evaluation of the court's proceedings to ensure no error in the law was made.
- *Settlement.* An agreement made by the defendant and the plaintiff at any point in the proceedings to end the lawsuit; generally this is for a financial sum.

7. Describe the application of the following legal concepts to paramedic practice: pp. 116–117

A. *Scope of practice.* The paramedic's scope of practice is the range of medical duties and skills that one is allowed to perform as determined by state law or other regulating body. Paramedics may not perform interventions or administer drugs that are not within their scope of practice; performing medicine outside of the scope of practice can result in the loss of licensure/certification and lawsuits.

B. *Licensure and certification.* The terms *licensure* and *certification* are often used interchangeably in EMS across the country, but the two are quite different. When an individual meets pre-established qualifications required to participate in an activity, that individual becomes certified. Certification

©2013 Pearson Education, Inc.
Paramedic Care: Principles & Practice, Vol. 1, 4th Ed.

might be by a government body, but can also be provided by a professional organization such as the National Registry of Emergency Medical Technicians. Licensure, on the other hand, is a governmental process to control the practice in a given occupation, and is granted to those who meet established qualifications based on education and training.

C. *Motor vehicle laws*. Every state has its own unique set of motor vehicle laws specific to emergency vehicle operation. For example, in many states ambulances can operate with lights AND sirens, but not with just one of the two. Carefully following the state's motor vehicle laws helps provide protection should a collision occur while operating the ambulance; violating the laws increases liability.

D. *Mandatory reporting requirements*. Like teachers, camp counselors, and physicians, paramedics are a professional group that has been identified though laws in most states as individuals uniquely able to help protect those who cannot protect themselves. These laws state that when cases including negligence, abuse (spousal, child, elder, physical, emotional, etc.), assault, rape, and violence occur, the paramedic must report these incidents to law enforcement or another formal body. Many states have set up reporting hotlines to ease this process. Every state has different specific requirements for what must be reported, and to whom. It is very important to become familiar with the mandatory reporting laws in each state in which you practice; not only is reporting these cases a moral obligation, but in some states a paramedic can be held criminally and civilly liable for failing to report the case.

E. *Legal protections for the paramedic*. Without a doubt, the best legal protection for any paramedic is to do the right thing in the patient's best interest 100 percent of the time. Unfortunately, paramedics often find themselves in less-than-ideal situations, which can include someone actually assaulting a paramedic, off-duty emergencies, and negative patient outcomes. In an effort to help promote the paramedic's ability to provide ideal care, some states have enacted laws to help provide additional protection. For example, some states have laws that make the assault of a paramedic a felony. Off-duty providers may be protected by Good Samaritan laws, which afford immunity to those who have no duty to act and offer care at the scene of a medical emergency. It is important to note although that many states require off-duty EMS providers to render care should they observe a medical emergency happening, these laws make the Good Samaritan law invalid. Immunity is a specific protection from legal liability to government workers. In some states immunity is extended to public service workers (public EMS model) when they are performing their jobs. Immunity does not protect anyone working for private, hospital, or other nongovernmental EMS systems.

F. *Employment laws*. Paramedics are protected by their individual state's employment laws that define employee and employer relationships. Employment laws range from defining fair wages and work conditions to workers' compensation and equal opportunities for employment. Some important laws to be familiar with include the Americans with Disabilities Act, Title VII and its amendments, the Family Medical Leave Act, the Fair Labor Standards Act, the Occupational Safety and Health Act, and the Ryan White CARE Act.

8. Given a scenario, determine whether or not the elements necessary for a claim of negligence are present. pp. 117–118

For a paramedic to be found negligent, the plaintiff must establish that the paramedic had a duty to act, that he breached that duty (did not provide the accepted standard of care), that the patient suffered damages, and that those damages were a result of the paramedic's actions.

All four elements must exist before negligence can be proven. The duty to act is the direct or indirect responsibility to provide the patient with care. Breach of duty is the failure to meet the standard of care associated with the patient's needs. Damages are the actual physical, psychological, or financial harm suffered by the patient. Proximate cause means that the paramedic's action or inaction directly caused or worsened the harm suffered by the patient.

9. Describe the paramedic's protections against a claim of negligence. p. 119

Actions that may help prevent charges of negligence include regular participation in education, training, and continuing education programs. Other protections include the use of on-line and off-line medical direction when appropriate; ensuring that all documentation is accurate, thorough, and objective; observing patient confidentiality; having a professional attitude and demeanor; acting in good faith; and using common sense.

In some situations, paramedics may also be protected from negligence by a Good Samaritan law, governmental immunity, or the statute of limitations. Each state has a different statute of limitations, which states that a lawsuit must be initiated within a specified time frame following the event in question.

10. Describe the special liability situations related to: p. 120

A. *Medical direction.* Should a paramedic be sued for his patient care, the off-line medical director may also be sued if he is found to have failed to have established proper protocols, performed quality assurance, or have breached his supervisory duties. An on-line medical director may also be sued if he ordered inappropriate interventions, denied needed interventions, or re-directed the ambulance to a facility that ultimately could not care for the patient.

B. *Borrowed servant doctrine.* Paramedics work as a part of a prehospital team. When working with a provider with less training or experience, it is the paramedic's responsibility to make sure that all skills and interventions are performed appropriately. This is particularly important at a scene with providers from multiple agencies. Should someone perform an intervention inappropriately while a paramedic is supervising the patient care, that paramedic can be held liable for a less-qualified individual's negligence under the borrowed servant doctrine.

C. *Civil rights.* Failing to provide proper and needed patient care because of a patient's race, creed, color, gender, national origin, sexual orientation, known disease state, or age is a violation of a patient's civil rights and may lead to a lawsuit.

D. *Off-duty practice.* Paramedics providing medical care when not on duty may only provide basic life-support interventions, such as stopping bleeding, CPR, spine stabilization, foreign body airway obstruction relief, and so forth. Providing advanced interventions without direct physician oversight (off-line medical direction) opens up the paramedic to lawsuits.

E. *Airway issues.* Proper airway management does not mean regular placement of an endotracheal tube. Rather, proper airway management means assuring a patent passageway for the entry of oxygen and the exit of carbon dioxide. Securing an airway may be performed with BLS or advanced interventions. When electing to perform endotracheal intubation, remember that it is a highly invasive skill with high risks. Whenever any advanced airway is placed, constantly re-confirm its patency. Failing to recognize a misplaced advanced airway can result in the loss of the right to practice in many states.

F. *Restraint issues.* The use of restraints is prudent and medically acceptable when they are needed to ensure that certain patients are kept safe from themselves and to keep medical providers safe from specific patients as well. Most hospitals have very clearly written restraint policies that specify what type of restraints may be used, when, and on which patients. These policies also define the ongoing monitoring required for the patient and the need for restraints. The best protection against negligence complaints regarding prehospital restraint application is through the development of careful training and policies regarding the use of both physical and chemical restraints. Take the time to learn established acceptable restraint practices rather than improvising your own in the moment of need.

11. Take measures to protect patients' confidentiality and privacy and comply with HIPPA. p. 121

Through their involvement in patient care, paramedics learn sensitive information about the patients treated. To encourage patients to continue to divulge this information, paramedics must respect its confidential nature and divulge it only to those with a need to know. Information regarding a patient may be released to those continuing care, in accordance with the patient's consent to release information, as required by law, and as necessary for billing purposes. The 1996 Health Insurance Portability and Accountability Act (HIPPA) increased the protective layers patients have for their personal information. The act also created rules requiring EMS agencies to take intentional measures to prevent the accidental (unauthorized) release of the patient's protected health information. To be HIPPA compliant, all EMS providers must receive consent from patients to share their personal information with hospitals and with insurance companies in order to ensure proper continued medical care and proper billing, respectively. When protected patient information is accidently distributed, HIPPA also requires that the patient be notified of the privacy breach and advised of what information was shared and with whom.

12. **Avoid written or spoken statements that could lead to a claim of defamation.** pp. 121–122

Imagine yourself at a motor vehicle crash where a 25-year-old male patient has rolled his vehicle several times in a small community. He is awake but confused and seems slightly combative. In addition, there is a strong odor of alcohol everywhere, with several broken liquor bottles in the back. During transport to the hospital you report: "we are transporting a 25-year-old heavily intoxicated male who was the driver of a vehicle that rolled at a high speed. It is difficult to tell if he has a head injury or if he is just drunk, which is making obtaining vital signs difficult." Upon arrival at the emergency department you transfer care to the trauma team, complete a report, and return to service.

Several months later, you receive notice of a lawsuit for slander. The same patient from the accident is suing you for defamation of character for stating he was a drunk driver. Apparently, the patient's blood alcohol level was zero and he had a blood sugar of 31. He could understand what you were saying but was not responding well enough to tell you about his diabetes. Unfortunately, everyone with a scanner heard that report you gave that stated he was driving and was "heavily intoxicated." He did have liquor bottles in the car, which shattered in the accident, spilling alcohol on him. The alcohol was for a party he was going to be hosting at his home.

It is easy to make small assumptions that can turn into large problems. To avoid potential defamation lawsuits, be sure to always stick to the facts whenever discussing a patient or when writing a report. For example it is OK to document "there is the smell of alcohol on the breath," but not "the patient is drunk."

13. **Given a variety of scenarios, select the type of patient consent that applies.** pp. 122–123

When a patient summons an ambulance, that action suggests that he is asking for help and consenting to treatment. However, a paramedic is obligated to explain what he is going to do to and for the patient and why he is going to do it. The paramedic must also determine if the patient is alert, oriented, and rational enough to make a competent decision to accept or refuse care. If the patient is not able to make a rational decision regarding care, the paramedic may need to invoke implied consent. If the patient is a minor and the legal parent or guardian cannot be reached, consent is assumed (implied consent).

14. **Given a variety of scenarios, manage withdrawal of consent and refusal of consent situations.** p. 123

When a patient refuses care, paramedics must ensure and document the following: the patient was legally able and competent to make the decision; the need for care and potential consequences of refusing care were explained; on-line medical direction was consulted (as needed); the patient was directed to see his own physician; and the patient was directed to call the ambulance if the symptoms return or get worse. The refusal form should be signed by the patient and either a family member or a police officer. If the patient refuses to sign a refusal of treatment form, then have his refusal witnessed by a family member or police officer.

15. **Given a variety of scenarios, manage problem patients.** p. 124

Imagine being called to the home of an 18-year-old female whose frantic parents called 911 after they found reason to believe their daughter may have ingested several pills. Everyone is crying, and the 18-year-old patient has no interest in being evaluated by paramedics. Despite being distraught, she seems to be alert and oriented. However, her parents insist she needs to be evaluated; in addition, there is an empty bottle of acetaminophen in a garbage can.

This situation presents a true dilemma. On the surface, if the patient is awake and oriented, she has a legal right to refuse care. However, if this was a suicide attempt, she loses that legal right in many states. The best way to deal with patients who may be potentially ill or injured, who are resistant to care, is to take the time to build a rapport. Establish that you are in no rush to leave and that you are there to make sure the patient is truly OK. Speak with such patients in a semi-private location, ask them to explain their situation in their terms, and repeat it back to them to show you understand. After understanding their situation, present them options that include allowing you to evaluate them but that avoid any threats, such as having them arrested. Explain to them in detail any risks associated with the problem at hand, and tell them how your and a physician's management can help mitigate those risks.

16. Maintain professional boundaries.

One of the hallmarks of a professional is being able to distinguish between acceptable and unacceptable practices related to the profession at hand. There are many important professional boundaries between paramedics, their patients, and other medical professionals. In order to help prevent a breach of a professional boundary it is important to maintain a vigilant effort to avoid becoming excessively tired, becoming seduced, and being unprepared for the work at hand.

17. Avoid situations that could lead to claims of abandonment, assault, battery, false imprisonment, and excessive force.

p. 126

Paramedics may face claims of abandonment when patient care is terminated without transferring it to another properly trained provider and patient care is still needed or wanted. This could occur should a chest pain patient be triaged to a BLS ambulance and the patient is discovered later to be experiencing a heart attack. Abandonment could also occur at a car accident if every patient is not evaluated appropriately. Imagine a vehicle full of people and one person saying "I think we are all OK," and as a result the ambulance departing the scene. If someone in that car was actually injured and was never evaluated, the paramedics on scene might be guilty of abandoning those individuals. To avoid abandonment, always provide diligent care, perform thorough assessments, and always offer patients an opportunity to be transported to the hospital.

Providing an assessment or initiating care on a patient without his consent is battery. Avoid battery by always obtaining consent for assessments and care. Assault can occur when specific treatments are threatened, such as a large IV for a scared child or threatening arrest if transport is not accepted. Respect people's wishes to refuse patient care or specific interventions. Although the risks of not having an intervention must be explained, it is never acceptable to threaten patients.

Forcing transport against a patient's wishes, even when it is ordered by a physician, is false imprisonment. To avoid false imprisonment charges, be sure to gain the patient's permission for transport in addition to consent for patient care. At times, certain patients may have had their rights to refuse transport taken away from them. These patient groups include some psychiatric patients, state and federal prisoners, and those with diagnosed disease who have permanently impaired cognition. In these situations, always be sure to have the paperwork showing who has the legal authority over the patient available prior to initiating transport.

Avoid the use of excessive force by being gentle and respectful with patients at all times. The amount of force used is a particular worry when managing combative or restrained patients. Too much force may be considered assault or battery. If force is ever needed to control or restrain a patient, only utilize it under the supervision of a police officer or a medical director.

18. Given a variety of scenarios, manage situations involving advance directives (including Do Not Resuscitate orders), organ donation, and decisions to withhold or terminate resuscitation.

pp. 126–130

Advance directives permit the patient to define what care he would desire should he become incapacitated and unable to express specifics about his own patient care. Advance directives include Do Not Resuscitate (DNR) orders, which limit care actions that can be taken should the patient go into cardiac or respiratory arrest. DNR orders have no impact on patient care until the respiratory effort or pulse cease. They are by no means a "do not treat." Living wills are legal documents that also prescribe the care a patient may receive should he be unable to communicate his personal wishes, including his desire to donate organs and to die at home or elsewhere. State statutes usually define the authority of DNRs, living wills, and other advance directives. It is essential to be familiar with the advance directive laws in your own state. Many states include prehospital care in some form of advanced directives but also require the advanced directive to be present at the time patient care is provided.

When presented with a patient who is a possible organ donor, it is essential for the paramedic to maintain adequate perfusion of that organ to ensure its viability. Employ resuscitation procedures, including fluid therapy, cardiac compressions, and ventilation, and notify the medical direction physician that you are transporting a possible organ donor.

©2013 Pearson Education, Inc.
Paramedic Care: Principles & Practice, Vol. 1, 4th Ed.

19. **Take appropriate actions to avoid destroying evidence at potential crime scenes.** p. 130

Your responsibility at the crime scene is first to ensure your safety and that of your patient and then to ensure the health of the victim (your patient). If the patient is not obviously dead, initiate resuscitation and care directed at his injuries. Limit any movement of articles around the patient and at the scene and, if possible, document what you moved and from what location you moved it. Do not cut through clothing where objects entered the body; remove the clothing without cutting it, or cut around the openings.

20. **Explain the elements of excellent documentation.** p. 131

Documentation establishes what was found and what was done at the emergency scene. It must be completed promptly, thoroughly, objectively, and accurately. At the same time, the confidentiality of the information obtained must be maintained. The documentation will become a part of the patient's medical record and help guide continuing patient care. It will also become a record of what you did at the emergency scene and during transport should your actions ever come into question. It may also become a legal document in a court of law when someone feels he has been injured (damaged) by someone else.

A patient care report must be completed in a timely manner, must be thorough, must be objective, must be accurate, and must ensure patient confidentiality to be an effective legal document.

Incomplete, inaccurate, subjective, or sloppy patient care reports suggest that patient care was incomplete, inaccurate, or sloppy or that your attention to the needs of the patient was not in keeping with your duty to act. Any modifications in the report, if not fully disclosed, suggest that you made an error and tried to cover it up.

Case Study Review

Reread the case study on pages 113−114 in Paramedic Care: Introduction to Paramedicine; *then, read the following discussion.*

This case study demonstrates the type of legal dilemma that many paramedics may encounter during their EMS responses.

The paramedics of EMS 117 are presented with a patient who is behaving bizarrely just before she becomes unconscious. They treat her, assuming that if she were conscious and alert she would recognize her need for treatment and consent to it (implied consent). Once she becomes conscious, she exercises her right to refuse treatment. The paramedics assess her and determine that she is able to make a rational decision and honor that decision. They recommend that she eat immediately to raise her glucose level and see her physician at the earliest opportunity. Although all of these actions seem reasonable, the paramedics are still exposed to legal responsibility for what happens to their patient after their care and release. In this case, their legal responsibility rises because the police suspected intoxication, and upon the patient's release there was still no confirmation that the patient had not been drinking.

Some responsibility may fall upon the paramedics should their patient not obtain something to eat, suffer a later drop in blood-glucose level, and injure herself or others while driving. It is essential that the paramedics carefully explain to the patient that she was driving erratically and appeared intoxicated. They must identify that if she does not obtain something to eat, this behavior may occur again and cause her to do harm to herself or others. They should also explain that this incident indicates the need for a medical evaluation of her condition to ensure that episodes like it do not occur again. She truly needs to see a physician immediately, and her refusal of transport to the hospital is against their expert advice.

The paramedics will further protect themselves by thoroughly documenting the incident. They must carefully identify what their assessment revealed and their reasons for administering dextrose. They must identify the results of their care (the patient becoming alert and oriented) and her subsequent refusal of further care. They must document that they encouraged her to go to the hospital with them and receive evaluation by a physician and that, when she refused, they had her speak with an on-line medical direction physician. In addition, the paramedics should document their advising her to obtain food immediately and to see her physician at the earliest opportunity. Her agreement to go to the mini-mart and obtain food as well as her assurance that she has an appointment with her physician should also be documented. Finally, they must have her sign a "release-from-liability" form and document by what criteria they determined she was rational and able to make that decision.

In a situation of this type, a good working relationship with the police might be helpful. The woman was clearly driving while impaired and is likely to receive a moving violation from the officer. Indicating to him the risk of a later fall in glucose level (if she does not eat) and a return to her erratic behavior might cause him to encourage the patient to ride with the paramedics to the hospital.

Content Self-Evaluation

MULTIPLE CHOICE

_____ 1. The term *liability* best refers to
A. an illegal act.
B. legal responsibility.
C. an act of negligence.
D. civil responsibility.
E. responsibility for damages.

_____ 2. Ethical responsibilities are best described as
A. requirements of case law.
B. requirements of statute law.
C. standards of a profession.
D. personal feelings of right and wrong.
E. legal concepts of right and wrong.

_____ 3. Which type of law is also called statutory law?
A. Case law
B. Common law
C. Legislative law
D. Administrative law
E. Regulatory law

_____ 4. Criminal law is best described as dealing with
A. wrongs committed against society.
B. conflicts between two or more parties.
C. contract disputes.
D. negligence.
E. breaches of faith.

_____ 5. Which of the following is/are a component of a paramedic's scope of practice?
A. Protocols
B. System policies and procedures
C. On-line medical direction
D. Training and continuing education
E. All of the above

_____ 6. Which of the following is NOT a common mandatory reporting event?
A. Rape
B. Spousal abuse
C. Child abuse
D. A seizure episode
E. Animal bites

_____ 7. Governmental immunity is a likely protection for the paramedic working for a municipality.
A. True
B. False

_____ 8. The Ryan White CARE Act provides what protection to the paramedic?
A. It requires a notification system for contagious disease exposure.
B. It compensates EMS providers who contract AIDS.
C. It permits EMS review of any patient records.
D. It grants immunity to civil litigation in cases of ordinary negligence.
E. It defines the restraints permissible while treating a violent patient.

_____ 9. Which of the following is NOT one of the elements required to prove a charge of negligence against a paramedic?
A. Duty to act
B. Proximate cause
C. Actual damages suffered by the patient
D. Payment to the paramedic
E. Breach of duty

©2013 Pearson Education, Inc.
Paramedic Care: Principles & Practice, Vol. 1, 4th Ed.

10. Which of the following is a duty expected of the paramedic?
    A. To respond to the scene of an emergency
    B. To conform to the expected standard of care
    C. To provide care in accordance with the system's protocols
    D. To drive, or ensure the emergency vehicle is driven, appropriately
    E. All of the above

11. The degree of care, skill, and judgment that would be expected under like or similar circumstances by a similarly trained, reasonable paramedic is
    A. the duty to act.
    B. the scope of practice.
    C. the standard of care.
    D. a proximate cause.
    E. malfeasance.

12. *Res ipsa loquitur* is a legal term that refers to
    A. contributory negligence.
    B. immunity from prosecution.
    C. a matter that is self-evident.
    D. the victim's liability.
    E. the reliability of evidence.

13. Which of the following may protect a paramedic from charges of negligence?
    A. Good Samaritan statute
    B. Governmental immunity
    C. The statute of limitations
    D. Contributory negligence
    E. All of the above

14. Although many employers and agencies carry insurance coverage, it is a good idea for a paramedic to obtain personal coverage because the agency's coverage may be inadequate.
    A. True
    B. False

15. In many states, a paramedic would be guilty of practicing without a license if, while off duty, he performed advanced life-support skills outside his system of medical direction.
    A. True
    B. False

16. Which of the following is NOT an acceptable reason for the release of confidential patient information?
    A. Medical providers need it to care for the patient
    B. A judge has signed a court order demanding its release
    C. It is necessary for third-party billing
    D. Other paramedics, not on the call, have requested it
    E. The patient has made a written request for its release

17. The act of injuring an individual's character, name, or reputation by false written statements and with malicious intent is
    A. slander.
    B. breach of confidentiality.
    C. malfeasance.
    D. misfeasance.
    E. libel.

18. Before beginning to treat a patient, a paramedic must obtain expressed consent.
    A. True
    B. False

19. The type of consent that is given by the authority of a court is
    A. expressed.
    B. implied.
    C. involuntary.
    D. informed.
    E. common.

20. For a patient's consent to be informed, the patient must be told and understand
    A. the nature of the treatment.
    B. the necessity of the treatment.
    C. the risks of the treatment.
    D. the risks of refusing the treatment.
    E. all of the above.

21. Once a patient has given consent for treatment, he may not withdraw that consent.
- **A.** True
- **B.** False

22. A minor is usually considered someone under the age of
- **A.** 16.
- **B.** 18.
- **C.** 19.
- **D.** 21.
- **E.** 25.

23. Conditions that may define a person as an emancipated minor include being
- **A.** married.
- **B.** pregnant.
- **C.** a parent.
- **D.** a member of the armed forces.
- **E.** all of the above.

24. Once a patient has withdrawn his consent to care, it may be considered assault to encourage the patient to go to the hospital.
- **A.** True
- **B.** False

25. Which of the following is NOT an essential element in accepting a patient's refusal of care?
- **A.** The patient is conscious, alert, and competent.
- **B.** The patient is a minor.
- **C.** The patient is aware of the possible consequences of his decision.
- **D.** The patient has been advised that he may call again for help if necessary.
- **E.** The patient and/or a disinterested witness has signed a release-from-liability form.

26. Ideally, a police officer should respond to the scene of all problem patients and sign the patient-care report as a witness or, if the patient poses a threat to the paramedic, accompany the paramedic and patient to the hospital.
- **A.** True
- **B.** False

27. Ending a patient–caregiver relationship without providing the appropriate continuing care and without the patient's approval could be found to be
- **A.** battery.
- **B.** defamation.
- **C.** nonfeasance.
- **D.** abandonment.
- **E.** assault.

28. The unlawful act of touching another person without permission is
- **A.** assault.
- **B.** abandonment.
- **C.** battery.
- **D.** slander.
- **E.** libel.

29. Which of the flowing is an important question to ask yourself when considering the restraint of a patient?
- **A.** Does the patient need immediate treatment?
- **B.** Does the patient pose a threat to himself?
- **C.** Does the patient pose a threat to others?
- **D.** All of the above
- **E.** None of the above

30. If you need to use force to restrain a patient, it is best to involve law enforcement whenever possible.
- **A.** True
- **B.** False

31. Under what situation should a paramedic NOT begin resuscitation of a pulseless, nonbreathing patient?
- **A.** The patient is obviously dead.
- **B.** The patient has a valid DNR order.
- **C.** There is obvious tissue decomposition.

©2013 Pearson Education, Inc.
Paramedic Care: Principles & Practice, Vol. 1, 4th Ed.

    D. There is extreme dependent lividity.

    E. All of the above are correct.

_____ **32.** Do Not Resuscitate orders usually restrict care providers from

    A. performing CPR in case of cardiac arrest.

    B. administering oxygen to a patient with shortness of breath.

    C. initiating IV access and giving pain medications.

    D. leaving the scene until the coroner arrives.

    E. contacting medical direction.

_____ **33.** If there is any doubt about the authenticity or applicability of a DNR order, a paramedic should initiate resuscitation immediately.

    A. True

    B. False

_____ **34.** Which of the following statements is NOT true regarding a paramedic's responsibility at the crime scene?

    A. He should contact law enforcement officers if they are not on the scene.

    B. He should not enter the scene unless it is safe.

    C. His primary responsibility is to preserve the evidence at the scene.

    D. He should not disturb the scene unless it is necessary for patient care.

    E. He should document the movement of any item at the scene.

_____ **35.** Which of the following is NOT required when documenting a patient-care response?

    A. Completing documentation promptly

    B. Ensuring that documentation is accurate

    C. Ensuring that documentation is subjective

    D. Ensuring that patient confidentiality is maintained

    E. Ensuring that documentation is thorough

Special Project

See Crossword Puzzle on next page

Crossword Puzzle

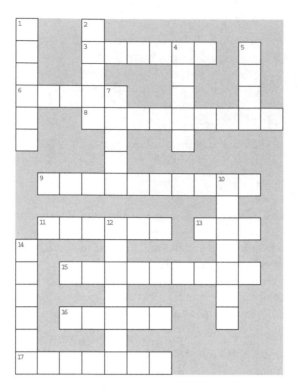

Across

3. Rules or standards of conduct that govern members of a profession
6. Right as determined by personal conscience
8. Legal responsibility
9. Deviation from the accepted standard of care
11. _____ will: document that allows a person to specify the kinds of treatment he would desire
13. _____ order: legal document indicating the life-sustaining measures to take during cardio-pulmonary arrest (abbr.)
15. _____ consent: communication from the patient indicating that he agrees to care
16. Component of a lawsuit in which both sides present testimony and evidence
17. Injuring a patient's character by false spoken statements

Down

1. _____ law: type of law derived from society's acceptance of customs and norms over time
2. Pertaining to the law
4. _____ law: division of the legal system that deals with noncriminal issues
5. A civil wrong committed by one individual against another
7. Injuring a patient's character by false written statements
10. A patient's permission to give care
12. _____ consent: type of permission to treat that is presumed from an otherwise incapacitated patient
14. Privileges that one is given by law and tradition

©2013 Pearson Education, Inc.
Paramedic Care: Principles & Practice, Vol. 1, 4th Ed.

Ethics in Paramedicine

Review of Chapter Objectives

After reading this chapter, you should be able to:

1. **Define key terms introduced in this chapter.**

   Knowing and being able to apply the key terms in each chapter is critical to understanding chapter concepts. Write the list of key terms. Then write the definition of each one in your own words. Check your understanding by confirming the definitions in the text glossary. Correct any misunderstandings. Create a study aid by writing each key term on the front of an index card and the definition on the back. Use the cards to quiz yourself or to have someone quiz you.

2. **Describe the relationship between ethics and morals, laws, and religion.**   pp. 136–137

   In general, the law takes a narrower and more specific look at behavior and identifies what is wrong in the eyes of society. Ethics takes a more general view of what is right or good behavior and tends to be viewed as more philosophical. Morals are a specific type of ethics based on social, religious, or personal standards of right and wrong.

   Laws and ethics are deeply entwined and entirely unique. No, that is not a trick statement. Consider, for example, a person's individual belief about his right to die via physician-assisted suicide (euthanasia) given a fatal disease. The laws in a given state will be very clear one way or the other on whether or not this is allowed. However, the ethical and moral discussions over this are endless. If a physician decides to support the patient's rights and personal wishes, how liable is this physician? Again the law will be clear, but again ethics overlap how the physician should be handled.

3. **Compare and contrast different approaches to ethical decision making.**   pp. 137–138

   Persons who practice ethical relativism believe that whatever someone perceives or truly believes to be right is ethically OK. However, ethical relativism rarely stands up in a true debate. For example, individuals practicing ethical relativism believed it was OK to place Japanese Americans in internment camps during World War II because they believed it was the best decision to protect the United States. By today's ethical standards, however, there is no acceptable reason to have done this.

   The golden rule of "do unto others as you would have them do unto you" is a great general rule to follow until ethical and legal laws blur. For example, in some states second-trimester abortions are illegal. However, some physicians may elect to perform them if a patient's health is threatened, claiming they might want the same for them if the roles were switched. In this case, ethics contradicts the law, and the right answer is unclear.

   Other different approaches to ethical decision making are full of advantages and disadvantages. These approaches include the Ten Commandments (Christian focused), also known as the deontological method; the consequentialism method; and faith-based practice. The challenge to all of these is balancing the patient's moral and ethical beliefs with our own as well as with the law.

4. Identify codes of ethics that serve to guide health care professionals, including EMS providers.   p. 138

EMT CODE OF ETHICS

Professional status as an Emergency Medical Technician-Paramedic is maintained and enriched by the willingness of the individual practitioner to accept and fulfill obligations to society, other medical professionals, and the profession of Emergency Medical Technician. As an Emergency Medical Technician at the basic level or an Emergency Medical Technician-Paramedic, I solemnly pledge myself to the following code of professional ethics:

- A fundamental responsibility to the Emergency Medical Technician is to conserve life, to alleviate suffering, to promote health, to do no harm, and to encourage the quality and equal availability of emergency medical care.
- The Emergency Medical Technician provides services based on human need, with respect for human dignity, unrestricted by consideration of nationality, race, creed, color, or status.
- The Emergency Medical Technician does not use professional knowledge and skills in any enterprise detrimental to the public well-being. The Emergency Medical Technician respects and holds in confidence all information of a confidential nature obtained in the course of professional work unless required by law to divulge such information.
- The Emergency Medical Technician, as a citizen, understands and upholds the law and performs the duties of citizenship; as a professional, the Emergency Medical Technician has the never-ending responsibility to work with concerned citizens and other health care professionals in promoting a high standard of emergency medical care to all people.
- The Emergency Medical Technician shall maintain professional competence and demonstrate concern for the competence of other members of the Emergency Medical Services health care team. An Emergency Medical Technician assumes responsibility in defining and upholding standards of professional practice and education.
- The Emergency Medical Technician assumes responsibility for individual professional actions and judgment, both in dependent and independent emergency functions, and knows and upholds the laws which affect the practice of the Emergency Medical Technician.
- The Emergency Medical Technician has the responsibility to be aware of and participate in matters of legislation affecting the Emergency Medical Technician and the Emergency Medical Services System.
- The Emergency Medical Technician adheres to standards of personal ethics which reflect credit upon the profession.
- Emergency Medical Technicians, or groups of Emergency Medical Technicians, who advertise professional services, do so in conformity with the dignity of the profession.
- The Emergency Medical Technician has an obligation to protect the public by not delegating to a person less qualified, any service which requires the professional competence of an Emergency Medical Technician.
- The Emergency Medical Technician will work harmoniously with and sustain confidence in Emergency Medical Technician associates, the nurse, the physician, and other members of the Emergency Medical Services health care team.
- The Emergency Medical Technician refuses to participate in unethical procedures, and assumes the responsibility to expose incompetence or unethical conduct of others to the appropriate authority in a proper and professional manner.

5. Explain the fundamental principles of ethics.   pp. 139–140

There are four fundamental principles/values of ethics. These principles are:
A. *Beneficence.* Beneficence is related to benevolence; beneficence means to do good, and benevolence is the desire to good.
B. *Maleficence. Maleficence* means to do harm, and when a paramedic or other medical professional performs a skill or intervention that causes actual harm to the patient, the provider can be charged in court with maleficence. Paramedics need to practice nonmalfticence, which means to not do harm.

©2013 Pearson Education, Inc.
Paramedic Care: Principles & Practice, Vol. 1, 4th Ed.

C. *Autonomy.* Competent adults have the right to autonomy, which is control over what happens to their own physical bodies. Paramedics cannot take away someone's autonomy, which is why consent must be obtained prior to providing patient care.

D. *Justice.* Justice means the delivery of equally fair care/judgment to everyone without consideration of sex, race, creed, ability to pay, background, or age.

6. **Given a variety of scenarios, recognize ethical dilemmas.**   **pp. 138–140**

Paramedic Smith provided the following patient report to St. Francis Hospital: "We are currently 10 minutes from your facility with a 62-year-old gentleman coming from his home who is complaining of difficulty breathing that has been getting worse since early this morning. Upon our arrival the patient had cyanosis at the lips and in the fingernail beds, was clammy, and had a productive cough. At this time we have administered a nebulizer treatment, have the patient on oxygen via nasal cannula, and have the following vital signs: pulse 124 and regular with a sinus rhythm on the heart monitor, respiratory rate 24 with some accessory muscle use, blood pressure 144/92; we do have an IV established at a KVO rate, his SpO_2 is 96 percent on 6 liters per minute of oxygen, and he has a tympanic fever of 101°F. Like I said, we have a 10-minute ETE; do you have any questions?" After this report a nurse came on the radio and replied: "We have no questions, but want you to take the patient off of oxygen so we can get a room air pulse oximetry reading when you get here."

How would you handle this request? What if St. Francis was your medical control hospital? What if the patient was not in respiratory distress after a nebulizer treatment?

7. **Given a variety of scenarios involving ethical dilemmas, take action you can defend on the basis of ethical principles of paramedicine and tests of ethical decisions.**   **pp. 140–141**

Determining how to respond to an ethical decision is not an easy task. When weighing a decision, it is important to consider beneficence, nonmaleficence, autonomy, and justice. Determine how making a decision one way or another affects each of these. For example, a decision to not give a blood transfusion to a Jehovah's Witness practitioner respects the patient's right to autonomy but does not reflect beneficence. When a decision cannot be made evaluating the four principles mentioned earlier, consider an impartiality test, a universalizability test, and an interpersonal justifiability test. These tests ask if a decision could be repeated if it affected you, affected other people in similar situations, and if the decision can be justified to others.

Case Study Review

Reread the case study on pages 135–136 in Paramedic Care: Introduction to Paramedicine; *then, read the following discussion.*

This case study shows the real potential for ethical dilemmas that can emerge during EMS responses. Here the care for the patient was not compromised because the paramedic caring for Mrs. Weinberg had equal or greater skill than the exchange student. The team worked together to accommodate the patient's medical needs and then the desires of Mrs. Weinberg.

What if Heinz was the paramedic of an EMT-B/Paramedic team? In the case described here, the patient needed only basic life support, but what if she needed IV fluids and pain medication? What if the case involved a female patient who had been physically abused or raped and was in need of advanced interventions? Can she request care from a female member of the team? Legally, the patient has the right to define his or her care (expressed consent). EMS members are obligated to accommodate the patient's requests, within legal limits, and if those requests diverge from good medical practice, they must carefully explain medical needs produced by the patient's condition and the risks of alternative therapy.

As ethics are defined as what society and professional peers expect, paramedics can be best guided by two principles: (1) provide the best medical care for the patient, and (2) then try to accommodate the patient's desires. Ethical decisions are not as black and white as most decisions in EMS, and system protocols do not address these situations. Often there is no one answer to an ethical question, and no two ethical situations are identical. However, paramedics who make decisions that do not meet the patient's medical needs or personal desires bring the profession into question and endanger its standing in the community.

Content Self-Evaluation

MULTIPLE CHOICE

_____ 1. Although ethical problems often have a legal aspect, most ethical problems are solved in the field and not in a courtroom.
   A. True
   B. False

_____ 2. Most codes of ethics provide specific guidance for the performance of the professional.
   A. True
   B. False

_____ 3. When faced with an ethical challenge, the best guiding question is which of the following?
   A. How would I like to be treated?
   B. What would the patient want?
   C. Which actions will account for the greatest good?
   D. What is in the best interest of the patient?
   E. What actions can I defend?

_____ 4. The term that means "desiring to do good" is
   A. benevolence.   D. autonomy.
   B. justice.   E. euphylanthropnia.
   C. beneficence.

_____ 5. The Latin phrase *primum non nocere* means
   A. "Do the best you can."
   B. "Avoid mistakes."
   C. "Maintain the patient's best interests."
   D. "First, do no harm."
   E. "Treat all patients fairly."

_____ 6. Which question best describes the impartiality test for analyzing an ethical situation?
   A. Can you justify this action to others?
   B. Would you want this procedure if you were in the patient's place?
   C. Would you want this procedure performed on a family member if he were in similar circumstances?
   D. Will you likely be questioned about the need for this procedure later?
   E. None of the above

_____ 7. When in doubt about the validity of a DNR order or the patient's desire to be resuscitated, you should
   A. begin resuscitation immediately.
   B. await arrival of the DNR to verify its validity.
   C. contact medical direction for advice before beginning resuscitation.
   D. do not resuscitate.
   E. begin with CPR and delay advanced interventions.

_____ 8. There are no circumstances in which it is appropriate to breach patient confidentiality.
   A. True
   B. False

©2013 Pearson Education, Inc.
Paramedic Care: Principles & Practice, Vol. 1, 4th Ed.

9. When presented with a patient who is enrolled in a health maintenance organization (HMO) whose policy states that the patient must be cared for at a member institution, you are responsible to act in the patient's best interest.
   A. True
   B. False

10. When presented with orders from a physician that do not comply with your protocols and that you believe are not in the patient's best interest, you should
   A. follow the physician's orders and report your concerns to the medical director.
   B. ask the physician to repeat or confirm the orders.
   C. ask the physician for an explanation of the orders.
   D. not follow the physician's orders.
   E. do all except A.

Special Project

Ethics and the Mass-Casualty Incident

Answer the following questions about the ethical dilemmas presented by mass-casualty incidents.

A. Define the normal approach to caring for a patient and explain why it differs at the disaster scene.

_____

_____

_____

_____

_____

_____

_____

_____

_____

_____

_____

_____

B. At a mass-casualty incident, a patient in cardiac arrest would not receive immediate care. Explain the reasoning behind this and the ethical dilemma it presents.

_____

_____

_____

_____

_____

_____

_____

EMS System Communications

Review of Chapter Objectives

After reading this chapter, you should be able to:

1. **Define key terms introduced in this chapter.**

   Knowing and being able to apply the key terms in each chapter is critical to understanding chapter concepts. Write the list of key terms. Then write the definition of each one in your own words. Check your understanding by confirming the definitions in the text glossary. Correct any misunderstandings. Create a study aid by writing each key term on the front of an index card and the definition on the back. Use the cards to quiz yourself or to have someone quiz you.

2. **Describe the benefit of effective EMS system communication to patient care.**   pp. 151–152

   Effective communications are essential to improving patient care. When the EMS system has quality communication systems, patient care benefits through early EMS notification, prearrival instructions initiating life-saving measures, streamlined intra-agency communications to limit scene time, and prepared equipment for patient care. There is also early activation of specialized hospital teams such as a trauma team, a stroke team, or a cardiac catheterization lab team.

3. **Discuss anticipated future trends in EMS system communication.**   p. 165

   The potential for future communication trends within EMS is exciting—already today paramedics can transmit 12-lead EKGs directly to emergency departments. In some areas on-line medical direction is no longer taking place via radio or phone, but rather through video communications where the physician can see exactly what is happening in the ambulance. Video communications such as this can help improve patient care by providing expert guidance to paramedics managing difficult cases. Another future communication trend may be the direct transmission of real-time data monitoring from cardiac monitors to deliver second-to-second updates on the patient's cardiac rhythm, pulse oximetry, blood pressure, end-tidal carbon dioxide levels, and temperature.

   Some systems are testing the prehospital use of portable ultrasound and CT devices where the information is transmitted directly to a physician for interpretation. Although the research in this area is still in its early stages, it provides real potential for early diagnosis of internal traumatic injuries and stroke.

4. **Identify the parties with whom you must communicate in the course of an EMS response and what you must communicate with each.**   pp. 151–152

   Throughout the evolution of an EMS response, paramedics must be prepared to effectively communicate with a variety of people. Proper preparation is important, because it is not wise to try to use the same terminology with everyone. For example, paramedics are unlikely to communicate with a physician and a 5-year-old patient in the same manner. Nor are paramedics likely to need to communicate the same information to a dispatch center as they might to the emergency department. Remember, communication is more than just spoken words—it includes tone of voice, mannerisms, facial expressions, and actions as well. Be prepared to communicate effectively with:

- The patient, who is likely to be anxious and distracted by his injury/illness
- Family members and bystanders, who may not have any medical understanding
- Personnel from other EMS agencies, fire departments, and police
- Physician, nurses, and other medical professionals at the emergency departments, physicians offices, and other health care locations
- The on-line medical director
- Communication specialists at the 911 center

5. Explain how the basic communication model applies to EMS communications.   p. 152

Any communication begins with the sender's idea or thought that the sender wishes to communicate. Once the thought is generated, a sender must decide how to encode the message through words, codes, tone of voice, actions, symbols, and so on. This encoded message is sent to a receiver, who must not only receive the encoded message, but also be able to decode, or translate, the message into terms he or she can understand. Once the receiver understands the message, the receiver typically acknowledges and communicates that he or she has received and understood the message.

This basic model is important in EMS, particularly when communicating with patients who do not know medical terminology. Thus when speaking with a patient, it is important to encode questions and statements in terms they understand. For example, you might not tell a patient "you are having a STEMI; we need to take you to the cath lab," as this language will not be understood. Instead, you might say "it seems your chest pain is caused by a heart attack; we need to take you to the hospital so a physician can correct it."

6. Describe factors that contribute to effective verbal communications.   pp. 152–153

There are many factors that contribute to effective verbal communications. When speaking with someone, it is important to use understandable words by avoiding jargon and local semantics. The use of "codes" and 10-codes may streamline communications within an organization, but can greatly confuse interdepartmental communications. For example, in one system a Code-4 may mean "we are OK," whereas in a different system, a Code-4 may mean that a patient is in cardiac arrest.

To help facilitate consistent effective communications, the Department of Homeland Security has established a program to help eliminate the use of coded messages during emergencies. Rather, it recommends the use of plain language for all radio traffic. Although the initial intent of this SafeCom program was for communications during large disasters, it is applicable to all organizations at all times because on nearly every EMS call in the country, paramedics have to communicate with many different groups.

7. Follow standard reporting procedures and format when communicating in the EMS system.   p. 153

When communicating within the system, it is important to follow a consistent and standardized format. This does two things. First, it allows for a regular approach to the information that is communicated from call to call, decreasing the opportunity to fail to communicate important information. Second, it standardizes what receivers can expect, so they are prepared and anticipate what information they will be receiving during each communication.

A standard patient report would be similar to the following: "General Hospital, Squad 54 … [go ahead 54] … Squad 54, paramedic Jones, we're en route to your facility from the scene of a 1-car roll over MVC with ejection with a 35-year-old female patient weighing approximately 200 pounds. The patient is complaining of shortness of breath and abdominal pain after being the ejected unbelted driver of the vehicle that rolled twice after hitting a tree at 55 mph. Her only medical history is two term live births; she is not pregnant at this time and on no medications. On exam she is awake but confused, does remember waking up after the accident, she has crepitus on the right lateral chest wall and tender-

©2013 Pearson Education, Inc.
Paramedic Care: Principles & Practice, Vol. 1, 4th Ed.

ness and rigidity over the right upper quadrant. At this time we have applied oxygen, have an 18-ga IV in place with normal saline running KVO. We are requesting orders for 50 micrograms of fentanyl. We currently have an ETE of 20 minutes. May we administer the fentanyl, and do you have any questions?"

8. Identify the uses of written communication in EMS, particularly those of the patient-care report (PCR). p. 154

The most common form of written communication in prehospital care is the patient-care report. This report is a legal representation of why specific care was or was not provided to a patient. Its contents, when legible, organized, and well put together, tell the story of what an EMS crew saw and did. Patient-care reports are invaluable tools. They permanently communicate why interventions were provided, are a source of reference for physicians and other hospital staff providing the patient's long-term care, are billing tools and educational tools, and are also used for quality assurance and research data collection.

9. Explain the purpose of the National EMS Information System (NEMSIS). p. 154

The NEMSIS database is a source to compile patient-care information from providers all over the country that can be used to truly establish best practices for EMS. Set data points are collected from every patient-care report generated, and this information is fed into the system. Looked at in aggregate, rather than each call alone, the database provides a true representation of how prehospital patient care is being provided all over the United States; the NEMSIS allows true national performance measurements that will allow benchmarking for future quality assurance projects.

10. Depict the sequence of communications in an EMS response. pp. 155–159

Miss Williams had not been feeling like herself all day. She felt more weak than normal and did not seem to have the energy she normally has. In an effort to get through her day, she kept working on her chores. She was taking a basket of laundry outside to hang on the line when her right side went limp. She quickly fell to the ground in the back yard. Fortunately her neighbors were outside with their children and saw her collapse, rapidly beginning the first step in an EMS response, *detection and citizen access*. Calling 911 on her cell phone Miss Williams's neighbor quickly activated EMS, and the dispatcher's *automated location indicator* was able to immediately provide an address for emergency responders. While simultaneously activating EMS, *emergency medical dispatch* information was provided to help Miss William's neighbor confirm that Miss Williams was breathing and had a pulse. *Prearrival instructions* were given to move Miss Williams onto her side, to protect her airway.

Once the first responders arrived on scene, they were able to communicate via radio to the responding paramedic unit that they had her on oxygen and provided vital signs. After their arrival and assessment, the paramedics suspected a stroke, and immediately began preparing Miss Williams for transport. As they left the scene they contacted their medical control physician on the phone, and explained to him their findings of right-sided weakness, an inability to speak, and hypertension. They also shared that they had confirmed Miss Williams had a normal blood sugar. They requested that the physician activate the stroke team, which the physician did, based on the information the paramedics shared. Once at the hospital, paramedics provided a *verbal patient report* to the receiving nurse and awaiting stroke team. They then completed their *written patient-care report* prior to returning into service.

11. Identify challenges and barriers to effective EMS system communication. pp. 152–153

The largest barrier to effective communication is the use of terminology that the sender may understand yet the receiver does not. This affects many areas of communications. For example, the use of 10-codes may be understood by a dispatcher and a paramedic; however, the same 10-codes are likely to not be understood by the patient, a medical control physician, or a nurse. Similarly, the physician and the paramedic may both understand medical terms such as STEMI or CVA; however, these terms again may not be understood by dispatch or the patient.

To avoid communication barriers, it is best to use simple terms and plain language during all communications. When plain language is used for communication, the messages are simplified and there is less room for confusion. This promotes group understanding and teamwork, and prevents the opportunity for safety concerns and medical errors.

12. Describe the responsibilities of EMS dispatchers. pp. 157–158

Communication specialists at a public safety access point (911 dispatch center) have several important functions. One of the first priorities is to identify the location and nature of an emergency. Once this is obtained they must activate the appropriate closest emergency responder, which is done based on call severity in a system known as priority dispatching. Simultaneously, they need to perform emergency medical dispatch to help individuals on the scene initiate any life-saving interventions that may be needed, including chest compressions, rescue breathing, and bleeding control.

For larger incidents the communication specialist must coordinate the response of multiple different agencies, such as police, fire, EMS, and emergency helicopters. Coordinated communication for all of these agencies is important to ensure that all providers know whom to expect at the scene, who else may need to be requested—such as additional ambulances—and when resources may be able to be cancelled.

The communications center also serves as the official recordkeeper for when 911 calls were initiated and when vehicles were dispatched, responding, and on scene. Because of their detailed recordkeeping, some 911 centers have the ability to advise responders when there have been multiple calls for the same address or when there is a history of violence at a location to help keep responders from entering a potentially unsafe location.

13. Demonstrate effective communications with dispatch, the medical direction physician, and the hospital staff receiving your hand-off report. pp. 158–159

Paramedics can demonstrate effective communication practices with their dispatch centers and medical control physicians by repeating back information they provide as well as any orders for patient care. This demonstrates that messages were not only received but also understood. In addition, if information was misinterpreted, the senders also are provided an opportunity to clarify their message.

When transferring patient care, provide a concise but thorough patient report at the time of patient hand-off. A good practice is to end the report by asking "what questions do you have?" This provides an opportunity for the receiver to ask to clarify and also sends a message that you have finished your message and also want to make sure it is understood.

14. Explain how communication and technology can contribute to situational awareness and a common operating picture. p. 160

For the past 40 years, EMS has been a service that identifies an emergency then looks for resources to address the issue. For example, first someone would arrive at the scene of an emergency, and then identify how many patients, and then request additional ambulances, and so on.

Through the use of advanced technologies, information can be linked from houses and vehicles to provide patient information, and 911 centers could have second-to-second statuses of all the response vehicles in their catchment. Many EMS systems already utilize software that allows paramedics to view what other ambulances are available in their service area at any given moment.

The installation of mobile data terminals in emergency response vehicles can allow a coordinated awareness of what other emergency vehicles are available. This knowledge can allow responders to know how long they may have to wait for additional resources, or have the knowledge going into an emergency that no other resources are available.

Imagine, for example, how differently a BLS ambulance crew may approach a call for an unresponsive patient if they were hoping an ALS unit might be available to respond, compared to if the EMTs knew before even arriving on scene that a hospital was going to be their most rapid access to ALS. This information could save valuable time during an emergency.

15. Describe the typical equipment, including advantages and disadvantages, and types of frequencies used in EMS system communication. pp. 160–165

Radio communication systems remain the primary form of communication for EMS systems across the country. There are several forms of radio systems in use today. The most common radio system is a simplex transmission system, which requires users to transmit and receive on a single radio frequency. Although this system utilizes the most basic equipment and is common throughout the country, it is limiting in its ability to effectively communicate because only one individual may speak at a time and a user must end his or her transmission before anyone else may transmit on the frequency.

Duplex transmission systems, like simplex systems, use radio frequencies for transmission. However, duplex systems utilize different frequencies for sending and receiving messages. By having two different channels, simultaneous communications are allowed (similar to speaking on a telephone); in addition, the duplex frequencies allow data transmission when not being used for voice transmissions. The biggest disadvantage to duplex systems is that with multiple people speaking at one time, it can be difficult to hear each individual. Multiplex systems were the next generation of duplex transmission systems. Although still having two communication frequencies, multiplex systems permit simultaneous voice and data transmission on a single frequency.

Many EMS systems found that with an increasing number of ambulances, dispatchers, fire services, and so forth, all attempting to communicate on the same frequencies, reliable communications was becoming difficult. This difficulty led to the development of trunked communication systems, where a "group" of radio frequencies, typically in the 800-MHz range, are bundled together into one system. When a user keys the communication group, a computer can then assign that use to a free channel in the group to relay a message. Upon completion of the message, the user releases the channel for another user. This grouping increases the ability for rapid communications for multiple users. However, due to the cost of the equipment for trunked systems, they are usually installed regionally. Without proper planning, groups who only come into the region on rare occasions—for example, ambulances from a neighboring county—may find themselves unable to communicate with a system with trunked communications.

Digital technology has become extremely common in many areas of life, and it is slowly working its way into EMS systems. When functioning well, digital technologies can integrate many operating systems and allow instantaneous transfers of information, including pertinent safety information, vehicle locations, and hospital statuses. Unfortunately, much of the digital technology is not designed for system stresses, such as during a disaster, and thus cannot be relied upon as a primary means of communications during major incidents. For example, cell phone systems are easily overrun and crash during evacuations and after storms. Although wireless technology is rapidly advancing, it needs to have its reliability increased prior to becoming an EMS mainstay.

16. Discuss the regulation of public safety communications. p. 168

All nongovernmental communication systems within the United States are controlled by the Federal Communications Commission (FCC). In 2008 the FCC established the Public Safety and Homeland Security Bureau, which now directly oversees EMS communications as well as other public-safety-related organizations. EMS communications are required, like all communications systems, to follow the established regulations and laws, which includes the use of frequency coordinators. The EMS frequency coordinator is the Internal Municipal Signal Association (IMSA).

17. Explain the importance of the ability to communicate effortlessly between multiple agencies and jurisdictions. p. 167

Major disasters, such as 9/11 and Hurricane Katrina, and smaller-scale events, such as multiple-vehicle car accidents when multiple agencies respond, have continuously emphasized the increased need for interagency communications systems. Too many emergency responders have been placed at risk for harm, or have not known where to respond and how to respond. This occurred because these responders were not able to effectively communicate with other agencies coordinating emergency efforts at a disaster.

Intra-agency communications needs have drawn enough attention that the National Emergency Communications Plan was developed in 2009 by the Office of Emergency Communications. At the same time, many states began developing their own statewide communications plans to coordinate the development of standardized effective communication systems throughout regions and across state lines.

Case Study Review

Reread the case study on pages 149–151 in Paramedic Care: Introduction to Paramedicine; *then, read the following discussion.*

This case study shows the real potential change in patient outcomes that can occur through the development and implementation of integrated communications systems both from a detection and EMS-activation perspective as well as from a patient management perspective.

This case study identifies some of the common and critical elements of communication essential to the emergency response. First, someone needs to recognize that an emergency exists (detection), and then activate the emergency response system (access). The dispatcher must then receive the call (call taking), determine its nature and seriousness, and dispatch the appropriate resources to deal with the problem (emergency response). The dispatcher determines the priority of the call by asking the caller a series of predetermined questions. The dispatcher, in addition, provides the caller with basic, approved first-aid steps to perform (prearrival instructions) until EMS reaches the scene to supply more comprehensive care. Additionally, the dispatcher also coordinates the response of any fire, police, rescue, or other service units needed to the scene (call coordination). Throughout this entire process the communication center records the pertinent information and times associated with the call for further review by the system administrator, the medical director, the quality improvement committee, researchers, or attorneys (incident recording).

Once at the scene and actively involved in patient care, paramedics contact medical direction to communicate the patient's condition and the care that has been initiated. This communication paints a clear picture of the patient they are treating. It may stimulate questions from the physician regarding the findings and patient care and may elicit orders for invasive actions or diversion from one hospital to a more appropriate receiving facility. When paramedics communicate with medical direction regarding orders, they use the echo procedure, repeating back the physician's orders word for word to ensure that both parties understand what is to be done.

The communications between paramedics and medical direction also enable the emergency department staff to prepare for the arrival of the patient (transfer communications). In this case, the patient's condition was critical and time was of the essence. Through effective communications the hospital was able to expedite the patient's movement toward the operating room.

This case is unique because it presents the same case with current communication systems and also presents with might happen if communications occurred with the most ideal technology available. Through streamlined and integrated communications systems, the accident's detection and access shift from delayed (until someone discovers it) to instantaneous. Technology allows a trained dispatcher to determine the precise location of the accident as well as the forces involved. These forces allow accurate prediction of injury severity and streamline the access to air-medical transportation to a trauma center. The integration of communications systems eliminates the need for individuals to repeat the same accident data each time someone new needs it, rather the information being electronically communicated to the responding units. Wireless technology also permitted Dr. Doyle to monitor the patient's vital signs before and during transport.

Although this technology seems to a degree based in fantasy, it is actually quite realistic. Individually, all of the technology is available—from patients carrying memory cards with personal data to cars having automatic crash notification, and even physicians viewing the scenes through paramedics and video. The present challenge with integrating all of these systems is designing communication systems that "talk" to one another and that are affordable for all aspects of the EMS system, including the ambulance services, communication centers, hospitals, and air-medical transport systems.

Content Self-Evaluation

MULTIPLE CHOICE

_____ 1. Essential participants in communications within the EMS system include
   A. the emergency medical dispatcher.
   B. the patient, his family, or bystanders.
   C. other responders, including police, fire, and other ambulance personnel.
   D. health care providers, including nurses, physicians, and medical direction physicians.
   E. all of the above.

_____ **2.** In general, although the use of codes shortens EMS communications, the lack of consistency of codes between EMS systems has led to coded messages being discouraged on a national level.
 A. True
 B. False

_____ **3.** A radio band is a
 A. series of radios that communicate with one another.
 B. pair of radio frequencies used for multiplexing.
 C. range of radio frequencies.
 D. pair of radio frequencies used for duplexing.
 E. none of the above.

_____ **4.** Use of proper terminology in both written and verbal communications will
 A. decrease the length of communications.
 B. increase the accuracy of communications.
 C. increase the clarity of communications.
 D. reduce the ambiguity in communications.
 E. all of the above.

_____ **5.** Features of the Enhanced 911 center include all of the following EXCEPT
 A. display of the caller's location.
 B. display of the caller's phone number.
 C. immediate call-back ability.
 D. a system of physician/ambulance interface.
 E. both B and C.

_____ **6.** The answering center for emergency calls, which then transfers them to the appropriate agency for dispatch, is the
 A. Enhanced 911 center.   **D.** emergency routing center.
 B. PSAP.   **E.** none of the above.
 C. GPS.

_____ **7.** Most current wireless phones do not provide the PSAP with the phone's location and call-back number.
 A. True.
 B. False.

_____ **8.** Which system may identify the exact location of a wireless phone?
 A. Geographic triangulation   **C.** Global positioning system
 B. Landline induction   **D.** Either A or C

_____ **9.** Terrestrial-based triangulation of a wireless phone's location is dependent on which of the following?
 A. Signal strength   **D.** The proximity of the PSAP
 B. Height of the wireless phone antenna   **E.** Both A and C
 C. Three towers receiving the signal

_____ **10.** The Enhanced 911 center may soon be notified of a vehicle collision, the forces involved, and its location through which of the following technological enhancements?
 A. ANI   **D.** PSAP
 B. ALI   **E.** None of the above
 C. AACN

_____ **11.** In the future, which of the following may be communicated to the dispatch center from a vehicle involved in a collision?
 A. The exact location of the incident
 B. A change in velocity of the collision
 C. The vehicle identification number
 D. The crash worthiness rating of the vehicle involved
 E. All of the above

©2013 Pearson Education, Inc.
Paramedic Care: Principles & Practice, Vol. 1, 4th Ed.   **CHAPTER 9** _EMS System Communications_   **83**

12. The system that uses standardized caller questioning to determine the level and type of response is
    A. priority dispatching.
    B. system status management.
    C. enhanced emergency medical dispatch.
    D. prearrival instructions packaging.
    E. dispatch triage.

13. The role of the modern-day emergency medical dispatcher includes
    A. priority dispatching.
    B. prearrival instructions.
    C. call coordinating.
    D. incident recording.
    E. all of the above.

14. The report that occurs as you transfer patient-care responsibilities to the emergency department staff must include
    A. chief complaint.
    B. assessment findings.
    C. care rendered.
    D. results of care.
    E. all of the above.

15. A radio system that transmits and receives on the same frequency is called
    A. simplex.
    B. duplex.
    C. triplex.
    D. multiplex.
    E. none of the above.

16. Which radio transmission design permits the receiver to interrupt the caller while the caller is talking?
    A. Simplex
    B. Duplex
    C. Multiplex
    D. Trunking
    E. None of the above

17. The radio system that uses a computer to determine and assign available frequencies is called
    A. simplex.
    B. duplex.
    C. multiplex.
    D. trunking.
    E. none of the above.

18. Advantages of cellular communications in EMS include all of the following EXCEPT
    A. duplex capability.
    B. direct physician/patient communication.
    C. ability to handle an unlimited number of calls.
    D. reduced online times.
    E. transmission of better ECG signals.

19. One of the paramedic's most important skills is gathering essential patient information, organizing it, and communicating it to the medical direction physician.
    A. True
    B. False

20. A standard format for transmitting patient information ensures all of the following EXCEPT
    A. communication efficiency.
    B. physician assimilation of patient condition information.
    C. completeness of medical information.
    D. easier use of multiplex signals.
    E. both A and C.

21. All of the following are appropriate for good EMS communications EXCEPT
    A. speaking close to the microphone.
    B. speaking across or directly into the microphone.
    C. talking in a normal tone of voice.
    D. speaking without emotion.
    E. taking time to explain everything in detail.

©2013 Pearson Education, Inc.
Paramedic Care: Principles & Practice, Vol. 1, 4th Ed.

22. It is important to press the microphone button for 1 second before speaking.
    A. True
    B. False

23. If the portable radio you are using is unable to transmit well from your location, attempt to
    A. move to higher ground.
    B. touch the antenna to something metal.
    C. move toward a window or away from structural steel.
    D. both A and C.
    E. none of the above.

24. The major difference between the medical and trauma patient reports is that the trauma format provides a description of the mechanism of injury and identifies suspected injuries.
    A. True
    B. False

25. The Federal Communications Commission is responsible for all of the following EXCEPT
    A. assigning licensing and radio frequencies.
    B. establishing technical standards for radio equipment.
    C. ensuring the proper use of medical terminology in radio communications.
    D. monitoring radio frequencies for proper use.
    E. spot-checking radio base stations for proper licensing records.

26. Which data collection tool is serving as a national resource for pooling EMS call data?
    A. FCC
    B. HHS
    C. NAEMT
    D. NEMSIS
    E. None of the above

27. The written patient-care report is used in all of the following areas EXCEPT
    A. in-hospital care.
    B. quality assurance.
    C. EMS research.
    D. billing.
    E. priority dispatching.

28. Throughout the course of an EMS call, paramedics are expected to have to communicate effectively with
    A. patients.
    B. bystanders.
    C. physicians.
    D. first responders.
    E. all of the above.

29. Which of the following terms would be an acceptable abbreviation or code understood by the majority of message receivers during EMS calls?
    A. DCAP-BTLS
    B. 10-97
    C. ETA
    D. Code pink
    E. "Tubed"

30. What was developed to help ensure that effective intra-agency communications can occur on a national level?
    A. NECP
    B. EMS for the Future
    C. OEC
    D. 10-codes
    E. National standard curriculum

31. The technology that may allow for real-time vital sign monitoring is
    A. multiplex.
    B. trunking.
    C. cellular communications.
    D. broadband.
    E. bandwidth.

32. Which of the following is a reason to consider medical control physician video access?
    A. Rural environment
    B. Portable imagery testing (ultrasound)
    C. Quality assurance for high-risk procedures
    D. All of the above.
    E. None of the above

33. What communications system is NOT recommended for the sharing of mission-critical communications?
- **A.** Written
- **B.** Face to face
- **C.** VHF radio
- **D.** Digital
- **E.** Duplex

Special Project

Documentation: Radio Report/Prehospital Care Report

The authoring of both the radio message to the receiving hospital and the written run report are two of the most important tasks you will perform as a paramedic. Read the following paragraphs, compose a radio message, and complete the run report for this call.

The Call

At 1515 hours, your ambulance, Unit 89, is paged out to an unconscious person at the local base-ball field on a very hot (97°F) Saturday. You are accompanied by Steve Phillips, an EMT, your partner for the day, and are en route by 1516.

You arrive on-scene at 1522 to find a young male collapsed at third base. He is unarousable and is perspiring heavily, and his skin is cool to the touch. The pillow under the boy's head (placed by bystanders) is removed, the patient's airway is clear, his breathing is adequate, and his pulse is rapid and bounding. One of the bystanders says the patient was playing ball and just collapsed. Another young bystander identifies himself as the patient's brother and states that "nothing like this has happened before." He says his brother is named Jim Thompson, is 13, and lives about a mile away.

The rest of the assessment reveals no signs of trauma. The assessment findings include blood pressure 136/98; pulse 92 and strong; normal sinus rhythm as revealed by the ECG; respirations 24 and normal in depth and pattern (at 1527). The boy responds to painful stimuli, but not to verbal commands or to his name. Pupils are noted to be equal and slow to react. Oxygen is applied at 12 L per minute by nonrebreather mask, and the patient is moved to the shade.

Receiving Hospital is contacted, and you call in the following report:

_____
_____
_____
_____
_____
_____
_____
_____
_____
_____
_____
_____

©2013 Pearson Education, Inc.
Paramedic Care: Principles & Practice, Vol. 1, 4th Ed.

Expected ETA at Receiving Hospital is 20 minutes.

Medical direction at Receiving Hospital, the closest facility, orders you to start an IV line with normal saline run just to keep open. You repeat the orders back to medical direction and then begin your care. Your first IV attempt on the right forearm is unsuccessful; the second attempt on the left forearm gets a flashback and infuses well. You retake vitals. The patient is now responding to verbal stimuli, the blood pressure is 134/96, pulse is 90, sinus rhythm is normal via ECG, respirations are 24. The patient is loaded on the stretcher at 1537 and moved to the ambulance.

You contact medical direction and provide the following update:

_____

_____

_____

_____

_____

_____

_____

_____

_____

_____

_____

ETA is 10 minutes.

En route, vital signs (at 1545) are blood pressure 132/90, normal sinus rhythm via ECG, pulse 88, respirations at 24. The patient is now conscious and alert, though he cannot remember the incident. The trip is uneventful, and you arrive at the hospital at 1557. You transfer the responsibility for the patient to the emergency physician and restock and wipe out the ambulance. You report back into service at 1615, grab a cup of coffee, and sit down at the hospital to write the run report.

Complete the run report on the following page from the information contained in the narrative of this call.

Compare the radio communication and run report form that you prepare against the example in the Answer Key section of this Workbook. As you make the comparison, keep in mind that there are many "correct" ways to communicate this body of information. Be sure that you have recorded the major points of your assessment and care and enough other material to describe the patient and his condition.

Date / /	Emergency Medical Services Run Report	Run # 911

Patient Information	Service Information	Times

Name:	Agency:	Rcvd :
Address:	Location:	Enrt :
City: St: Zip:	Call Origin:	Scne :
Age: Birth: / / Sex: [M][F]	Type: Emrg[ ] Non[ ] Trnsfr[ ]	LvSn :
Nature of Call:		ArHsp :
Chief Complaint:		InSv :

Description of Current Problem:

Medical Problems

Past		Present
[ ]	Cardiac	[ ]
[ ]	Stroke	[ ]
[ ]	Acute Abdomen	[ ]
[ ]	Diabetes	[ ]
[ ]	Psychiatric	[ ]
[ ]	Epilepsy	[ ]
[ ]	Drug/Alcohol	[ ]
[ ]	Poisoning	[ ]
[ ]	Allergy/Asthma	[ ]
[ ]	Syncope	[ ]
[ ]	Obstetrical	[ ]
[ ]	GYN	[ ]

Other:

Trauma Scr: Glasgow:

On-Scene Care:	First Aid:
	By Whom?

O₂@ L : Via   C-Collar :   S-Immob. :   Stretcher :

Allergies/Meds:	Past Med Hx:

Time	Pulse	Resp.	BP S/D	LOC	ECG
:	R: [r][i]	R: [s][l]	/	[a][v][p][u]	
Care/Comments:					
:	R: [r][i]	R: [s][l]	/	[a][v][p][u]	
Care/Comments:					
:	R: [r][i]	R: [s][l]	/	[a][v][p][u]	
Care/Comments:					
:	R: [r][i]	R: [s][l]	/	[a][v][p][u]	
Care/Comments:					

Destination:	Personnel:	Certification
Reason:[ ]pt [ ]Closest [ ]M.D. [ ]Other	1.	[P][E][O]
Contacted: [ ]Radio [ ]Tele [ ]Direct	2.	[P][E][O]
Ar Status: [ ]Better [ ]UnC [ ]Worse	3.	[P][E][O]

Documentation

Review of Chapter Objectives

After reading this chapter, you should be able to:

1. **Define key terms introduced in this chapter.**

   Knowing and being able to apply the key terms in each chapter is critical to understanding chapter concepts. Write the list of key terms. Then write the definition of each one in your own words. Check your understanding by confirming the definitions in the text glossary. Correct any misunderstandings. Create a study aid by writing each key term on the front of an index card and the definition on the back. Use the cards to quiz yourself or to have someone quiz you.

2. **Explain the purpose and goals of the patient-care report in EMS.**   **p. 173**

   The purpose of the prehospital patient-care report is to accurately document a thorough explanation of the assessment findings and medical care offered and provided during the interactions of a patient with the prehospital medical providers. This documentation is a permanent part of the patient's medical record and can influence his care for years.

       Proper, legible, and accurate documentation in a patient-care report is essential to help the report achieve its three primary goals:

   - To provide information to subsequent health care professionals about the patient and treatments provided in the prehospital setting
   - To provide essential information for proper billing of the patient
   - To provide a legal record of the call's circumstances

3. **Explain the importance of proper spelling, terminology, abbreviations, and acronyms, or as an alternative, plain English, in written documentation.**   **pp. 174–176**

   Medical terminology is the very precise and exact wording used to describe the human body and injuries or illnesses. Proper use of this terminology turns the PCR into a medical document. However, if terms are misspelled or misused, they may distract from the document and confuse the reader about the patient's condition and the care he has had or should receive. Carry a pocket dictionary, and use words only when you are sure of their spelling and their usage. The same holds true of medical abbreviations. They must be applied properly and have the same meaning to both the writer and the reader. EMS systems should use a standardized set of abbreviations and acronyms to ensure good and efficient documentation.

4. **Discuss the importance of accurate documentation of times and radio communications.**   **p. 176**

   Careful and accurate documentation of times is extremely important. Physicians, lawyers, quality assurance coordinators, and researchers all pay close attention to the times 911 calls took place, medicines that were administered, and when hospitals were notified, just to name a few aspects of documentation. When documenting times on a run report, be sure to always confirm that pertinent times align with those obtained or documented by the communication center. Documenting times that do not match those in the communications center can affect accuracy, calling other aspects of a PCR into question.

A good practice is to synchronize your watch with the communications center clocks at the beginning of every shift. This provides a reliable source for the times interventions were provided and medicines were administered. Imagine documenting an intervention time that was actually a time prior to when the communication center had your ambulance on scene!

Accurate documenting of radio communications is also important. Designated trauma centers and cardiac centers carefully monitor the response times of their specialized teams. These hospitals may utilize your patient-care reports to note when teams were activated to determine if they are responding appropriately.

5. **Given a series of patient-care reports, identify the elements of good communication.** pp. 182–185

Every patient-care report is going to be slightly different based on the patient's complaint and how the patient was managed. However, every well-written report has a few common elements. These elements include:

- Completeness and accuracy
- Legibility
- Absence of alterations (or properly documented addendums)
- Timely completion
- Evidence of professionalism
  - Absence of jargon
  - Absence of opinionated statements
  - Clear objectivity
  - Avoidance of libelous comments

6. **Given a variety of patient-care scenarios, write effective patient-care narratives using a standard format.** pp. 185–187

Well-prepared and well-structured narratives have a subjective section that identifies the patient's chief complaint and explains how the patient reports his present illness and prior medical history. Narratives continue with a factual and objective description of the exam findings and then the treatment provided. Although there are a variety of standard means for preparing a narrative—including a body system's approach, SOAP, CHART, and patient-management-focused narratives—the following is an example of a well-written narrative:

Squad 54 was dispatched to a residential address for reports of chest pain. Upon arrival at 0543 the EMS crew found a 54-year-old female patient in her nightgown seated on her couch awake and alert but anxious. She reports that she was awoken at 0500 with 7 out of 10 chest heaviness that radiates into her left arm and jaw that does not change upon exertion and deep respiration. She also reports that this discomfort is similar to what she experienced when she had a previous heart attack four years ago. The patient continues that she also has a history of hypertension and diet-controlled diabetes. She is requesting transport to St. Sebastian's hospital.

Upon exam the patient is awake and oriented but appears anxious. She denies dizziness or vertigo. Pupils are equal and reactive, airway is patent and self-maintained, there is JVD as the patient sits upright. Lung sounds are clear bilaterally; she does have chest pain as described above; it does not change upon palpation. Abdomen is soft and not tender; the patient states she is nauseous but has not vomited. Her extremities are intact with 1+ pedal edema noted, and strong distal pulses are present in all four extremities. Her skin is slightly pale but warm and she is clammy.

Oxygen was provided at 2 LPM via nasal cannula, vitals were obtained at 0550, and a 12-lead EKG was performed showing a sinus rhythm at a rate of 94 beats per minute with ST segment elevation in leads II, III, aVF. The patient was rapidly moved to the ambulance via stretcher secured x5 seat belts and emergent transport was initiated to St. Sebastian's. During transport a cardiac alert was given at 0558 with a 25-min ETE, an IV was established with an 18 ga in the left forearm with normal saline infusing KVO without signs of infiltration. Oral ASA 324 mg was administered at 0600 and 0.4 mg nitroglycerine SL was administered at 0603. Following the nitroglycerine, vital signs were repeated without changes and the patient remains hypertensive at 184/112. Zofran 4-mg IV was administered for her nausea 0605 and morphine 2-mg IV was given for her pain at 0606. The nitroglycerine 0.4-mg SL was repeated at 0608 and 0613 with the patient's pain reduced to 2 out of 10 at 0618. The 12-lead EKG was repeated at 0619 without any changes noted from the initial 12-lead EKG. She remained without other changes during the remainder of the transport and patient care was transferred to the ED staff upon arrival in Cardiac Room 1 with full report and the patient's medications with the patient still awake and oriented.

7. Discuss the differences in documentation for special situations such as refusals of care and mass-casualty incidents.   **pp. 189–190**

Often a multiple-casualty situation calls for an atypical EMS response and unusual documentation procedures. Care providers rarely stay with a patient from the beginning to the end of prehospital care, and the time spent at a patient's side is very much at a premium. Therefore, documentation must be efficient and incremental. Document your assessment findings and any interventions you perform at the patient's side quickly and clearly. Many agencies or systems have their own forms, such as triage tags, that simply document the procedure. Because triage tags have become standard across the country, they are considered a permanent part of the medical record and often no additional information, other than what is on a completely filled out triage tag, is needed to document prehospital care during a multiple-casualty incident.

Be careful in the documentation of a patient who refuses care or transport. Although a conscious and mentally competent patient has the right to refuse care, his doing so may pose legal problems for care providers. Document the nature and severity of the patient's injuries, any care you offered, and any care the patient refused, and document carefully the assessment criteria you used to determine the patient was capable of making the decision to refuse care or transport. Also document the patient's reasons for refusing care and your efforts to convince the patient to change his mind. If possible, have the refusal of care and your explanation to the patient of the consequences of care refusal signed by the patient and witnessed by family, bystanders, or police. Advise the patient to seek other medical help, such as a family physician, and to call EMS again if he changes his mind or if his condition worsens.

8. Predict the consequences of inappropriate documentation.   **p. 191**

A legible, complete, and accurate PCR is essential to call documentation. The information in it must be easy to read thanks to both good penmanship and conscientious attention to detail. The report must describe all the pertinent information gathered at the scene and en route to the hospital, as well as all actions taken by you and others in the care of the patient. Failure to create a thorough, readable PCR reduces the information available to other caregivers and may reduce their ability to provide effective care. The document you produce also reflects on your ability to provide assessment and care of your patient and your professionalism in general.

9. Discuss the benefits and drawbacks of electronic patient-care reports as compared to paper patient-care reports.   **pp. 191–192**

There are many benefits in transitioning from paper to electronic documenting of patient care. The ePCR is available in many styles, and although each program has it owns advantages and disadvantages, all of the electronic charting programs as a whole allow for a simplified and more consistent standard for communicating information with hospitals and also for billing and quality assurance. Many of the charting systems also have built-in quality assurance programs that make it easier to perform data collection and data analysis. Illegibility is eliminated with electronic charting, as everything is typed into the system. Additionally, misspellings can be avoided by taking advantage of spell-checking software within the program. Each charting system can be personalized for the services using the program to allow for every ambulance service to add additionally needed features or eliminate unnecessary features. Many charting systems can also be integrated to communicate with dispatch and billing software to ensure that information is consistently and accurately transmitted between departments.

Even with all of these advantages, there are some disadvantages to electronic charting. The most significant disadvantage is the initial start-up cost and training. Not only must the software be purchased, but computers also need to be purchased to perform the charting on. Over time, software upgrades will require additional purchases. Another disadvantage is retraining staff on an entire system with a new charting style. These disadvantages, though, can be overcome, as initial costs can be mitigated though long-term quality assurance growth and improved performance, and a more standardized approach to documentation can improve billing practices as well as reduce an organization's risks from lawsuits.

Case Study Review

Reread the case study on page 172 in Paramedic Care: Introduction to Paramedicine; *then, read the following discussion.*

This case study identifies some of the important considerations regarding the prehospital care report and its potential to support (or incriminate) a care provider who is called into a court of law. The scenario emphasizes the importance of good documentation.

We seldom realize the importance of the role of others in our prehospital documentation. In this case study, Tom Brewster is surprised when, three years after a call, he is summoned to give a legal deposition about it. Although this example speaks to legal reasons for review of documentation, Tom might just as well have been asked about the quickness of the ambulance response, the time he and his crew spent on scene, or specific aspects of the care he provided. Oftentimes it is the information that is absent from a patient-care report that investigators ask most about. Thus, the more information included in a report, the better the result can be when asked about a call years after it originally took place. Although attorneys may represent the most feared interrogators to most paramedics, the EMS system medical director, quality improvement personnel, or administrative personnel might also ask for details of an incident that took place months or years in the past. For these reasons, your accurate and thorough documentation of the emergency scene and the assessment and care you provide is of great importance to you and your service.

Tom was asked about his recall of the events of the call and the comments made by the patient. His prehosptial care report provided enough information to prompt Tom to remember the incident, the patient, and the care he gave. He was fortunate that his documentation provided this information and that he could piece together the events of that response. It is likely that the patient's attorney would challenge Tom's recall after three years. Documentation of the patient's statement that he "fell asleep" would be a factor critical in determining the reason for the crash (ruling out medical causes). Tom was apparently thorough in gathering the patient history and recording it on the PCR, because he was able to recall that there was no history of either diabetes or heart disease. Tom further benefited from performing a routine but complete patient assessment, including glucose testing and ECG monitoring.

This case study emphasizes the importance of preparing a prehospital care report that describes exactly what happened and exactly what was done. Had Tom used sloppy penmanship or subjective statements or failed to provide complete information, the patient's attorney would have been able to challenge Tom's objectivity and accuracy. As things stood, the report supported Tom's recall and evaluation of the patient's condition.

Consider Tom's partner: would he or she recall the events exactly as Tom did? What would he or she state compared to Tom if their testimonies were compared side by side? How does your partner recall events as compared to you? Do you and your partner routinely read one another's reports?

Content Self-Evaluation

MULTIPLE CHOICE

_____ 1. The prehospital care report is likely to be reviewed by which of the following?
    A. Researchers
    B. EMS administrators
    C. Lawyers
    D. Medical professionals
    E. All of the above

2. Which of the following is NOT an appropriate purpose for reviewing a prehospital care report?
   A. To identify a chronological account of the patient's mental status
   B. To learn about what calls other paramedics had
   C. To help detect patient improvement or deterioration
   D. To identify what bystanders and family said at the scene
   E. To determine baseline assessment findings

3. The prehospital care report may yield information that the quality improvement committee may use to identify problems with individual paramedics or with the EMS system.
   A. True
   B. False

4. The prehospital care report should contain all of the following EXCEPT
   A. a description of your patient's condition when you arrived.
   B. your opinions about the patient's attitude or social/economic situation.
   C. a description of your patient's condition after interventions.
   D. the medical status of your patient upon arrival at the emergency department.
   E. response time to the call.

5. If you have doubts about the spelling of a term when completing a PCR, use a phonetically close spelling; doing this may still convey the right meaning and will not reflect poorly on your professionalism.
   A. True
   B. False

6. Which of the following is NOT a time commonly recorded on the prehospital care report?
   A. Call received
   B. Dispatch time
   C. Arrival at the patient's side
   D. Arrival at the emergency department
   E. First physician contact time

7. Since your watch, the dispatch clock, and other timing devices are not often synchronized, it is important to record all times on the PCR from one clock or watch when possible or to indicate when different clocks were used.
   A. True
   B. False

8. Which of the following is NOT an example of a pertinent negative?
   A. No shortness of breath in a myocardial infarction patient
   B. No history of epilepsy in a seizing patient
   C. Clear breath sounds in a congestive heart failure patient
   D. A blood pressure of 90/60
   E. No jugular vein distension in a congestive heart failure patient

9. The recommended way of indicating the exact words spoken by a patient or bystander is to
   A. underline the passage.
   B. draw one line through the center of the word or passage.
   C. begin and end the passage with quotation marks.
   D. place the passage in parentheses.
   E. write the entire passage in capital letters.

10. All of the following describe good documentation EXCEPT
    A. complete.
    B. altered.
    C. accurate.
    D. objective.
    E. legible.

_____ 11. The PCR is created by the paramedic as a personal record of what happened at the scene and during transport, and thus its legibility to others is NOT important.
   A. True
   B. False

_____ 12. The benefit of check boxes on a prehospital care report is that they
   A. ensure that common information is recorded for every call.
   B. eliminate the need for a patient narrative.
   C. address every chief complaint.
   D. speed the completion of the narrative.
   E. all of the above.

_____ 13. When should the prehospital care report be completed?
   A. At the end of the day
   B. At the end of the duty shift
   C. Once back in quarters
   D. Shortly after leaving the hospital
   E. Upon or shortly after transferring patient care at the hospital

_____ 14. Whenever possible, have all members of your crew read or reread the prehospital care report before you submit it.
   A. True
   B. False

_____ 15. Which of the following is the best example of a subjective and possibly libelous statement?
   A. "The patient smelled of alcohol."
   B. "The patient walked with a staggering gait."
   C. "The patient used abusive language and spoke with slurred speech."
   D. "The patient was drunk and obnoxious."
   E. None of the above statements are subjective or libelous.

_____ 16. The management portion of your documentation should include which of the following?
   A. Any interventions   D. Changes in the patient's condition
   B. The results of ongoing assessments   E. All of the above
   C. The patient's condition when care is transferred at the emergency department

_____ 17. Which of the following is NOT a part of the subjective information recorded on the PCR?
   A. Vital signs   D. Past medical history
   B. Review of symptoms   E. None of the above
   C. Chief complaint

_____ 18. Which of the following is an element of the objective information recorded on the PCR?
   A. General impression of the patient   D. Results of any diagnostic tests
   B. Results of the physical exam   E. All of the above
   C. Vital signs

_____ 19. In obtaining a patient refusal against medical advice, it is important to
   A. determine that the patient is alert, oriented, and competent to make the decision.
   B. clearly explain to the patient the risks of not receiving care.
   C. confirm the patient understands the possible consequences of his decision.
   D. explain that if the condition worsens, the patient should call for the ambulance or otherwise seek immediate care.
   E. all of the above.

_____ 20. A disadvantage of electronic patient-care reporting is
   A. standardized reporting takes away creativity.
   B. quality assurance more easily identifies issues.
   C. the initial cost of the equipment.
   D. reports appear similar for every call.
   E. spelling errors can be reduced.

©2013 Pearson Education, Inc.
Paramedic Care: Principles & Practice, Vol. 1, 4th Ed.

Special Project

Documentation: Radio Report/Prehospital Care Report

The preparation of both the radio message to medical direction and writing of the written run report are two of the most important tasks you will perform as a paramedic. Read the following information, compose your initial and updated radio messages, and then complete the run report for this call.

The Call

At 1832, medic rescue Unit 21 is paged through dispatch and is en route to a one-car collision at the corner of Elm and Wildwood Lanes. One patient is reported unconscious, and the fire department is also en route. You and your partner, Mike Grailing (a paramedic), arrive with the ambulance at 1845 and find that there are wires down, fuel spilling from the gas tank, and window glass around the scene. Bystanders state that the car swerved wildly, then hit the power pole. You notice there are no skid marks. You stand by, awaiting arrival of the fire department and the securing of the scene.

Once the scene is safe, your partner employs a jaw-thrust with cervical precautions and applies cervical stabilization, while you apply the cervical collar (1850) and begin the assessment. You notice a break in the car's windshield and a small contusion on your patient's forehead. He is unconscious, has a strong pulse, and displays some respiratory wheezing and stridor. Assessment of the neck reveals a small welt but no other apparent injuries. The pupils are equal and reactive. Oxygen is administered at 12 L per minute via nonrebreather mask, the patient awakens, and initial vitals (including a respiratory rate of 30 with audible wheezes, blood pressure of 110/76, a strong pulse of 90, and oxygen saturation of 94 percent) are taken at 1852. The ECG displays normal sinus rhythm.

The patient awakens and asks, "What happened?" He states that he thinks he was stung by a bee. Two years ago he had a similar sting and reaction and has a kit at home that his physician prescribed for him. He is experiencing itching, and there are noticeable hives. He says he feels like "I have a lump in my throat."

Based upon protocol, you initiate the IV run TKO with lactated Ringer's solution in the right forearm using a 16-gauge over-the-catheter needle while the patient is being immobilized and moved to a long spine board.

Medical direction is contacted and you call in the following:

_____

_____

_____

_____

_____

_____

_____

_____

_____

_____

_____

_____

Orders for 0.3 mg epinephrine subcutaneously (1:1,000) and 50 mg Benadryl IM are received, and the medications are administered at 1855. Just prior to moving the patient to the ambulance, the patient is monitored and found to have the following vitals: blood pressure 118/88, pulse 78 strong and regular, respirations 20 and regular with clear breath sounds, an ECG showing normal sinus rhythm, and a pulse oximetry reading of 99 percent.

The patient history, which is taken at the scene and during transport, reveals that the patient's name is William Sobeski, his age is 28, and he lives at 2145 East Brookline Drive in the city of Rochester. The patient denies any allergy, except to bee stings. He was stung by a bee 2 years ago and was rushed to the emergency department because he "couldn't catch his breath." He denies any headache, visual disturbances, and numbness and tingling. He also denies taking any prescribed medications and has not eaten since noon. The patient requests Community Hospital because his sister works there. En route, vitals are blood pressure 122/78, pulse of 68 strong and regular, respirations 22 and regular, and a pulse oximetry reading of 98 percent, all taken at 1902.

Contact medical direction and provide the following update:

_____

_____

_____

_____

_____

_____

_____

_____

_____

_____

ETA is 10 minutes.

The final vitals, taken just before arrival, are blood pressure 122/80, pulse 86, oxygen saturation of 98 percent, and respirations 24 and regular with no wheezes. The ECG still displays normal sinus rhythm, and the patient is conscious and oriented. He states that the feeling of a lump in the throat is gone.

The trip is uneventful, and the patient is delivered to the emergency department at 1925. The patient care responsibilities are transferred to the staff, and the attending physician is given the final patient update. The vehicle is restocked and cleaned, and you are ready for service at 1955.

Using the information contained in this narrative, complete the run report on the next page.

©2013 Pearson Education, Inc.
Paramedic Care: Principles & Practice, Vol. 1, 4th Ed.

Date / /	Emergency Medical Services Run Report	Run # 911

Patient Information	Service Information	Times

Name:	Agency:	Rcvd :
Address:	Location:	Enrt :
City: St: Zip:	Call Origin:	Scne :
Age: Birth: / / Sex: [M][F]	Type: Emrg[ ] Non[ ] Trnsfr[ ]	LvSn :
Nature of Call:		ArHsp :
Chief Complaint:		InSv :

Description of Current Problem:

Medical Problems

Past		Present
[ ]	Cardiac	[ ]
[ ]	Stroke	[ ]
[ ]	Acute Abdomen	[ ]
[ ]	Diabetes	[ ]
[ ]	Psychiatric	[ ]
[ ]	Epilepsy	[ ]
[ ]	Drug/Alcohol	[ ]
[ ]	Poisoning	[ ]
[ ]	Allergy/Asthma	[ ]
[ ]	Syncope	[ ]
[ ]	Obstetrical	[ ]
[ ]	GYN	[ ]

Other:

Trauma Scr: Glasgow:

On-Scene Care:	First Aid:
	By Whom?

O₂ @ L : Via	C-Collar :	S-Immob. :	Stretcher :

Allergies/Meds:	Past Med Hx:

Time	Pulse	Resp.	BP S/D	LOC	ECG
:	R: [r][i]	R: [s][l]	/	[a][v][p][u]	
Care/Comments:					
:	R: [r][i]	R: [s][l]	/	[a][v][p][u]	
Care/Comments:					
:	R: [r][i]	R: [s][l]	/	[a][v][p][u]	
Care/Comments:					
:	R: [r][i]	R: [s][l]	/	[a][v][p][u]	
Care/Comments:					

Destination:	Personnel:	Certification
Reason:[ ]pt [ ]Closest [ ]M.D. [ ]Other	1.	[P][E][O]
Contacted: [ ]Radio [ ]Tele [ ]Direct	2.	[P][E][O]
Ar Status: [ ]Better [ ]UnC [ ]Worse	3.	[P][E][O]

INTRODUCTION TO PARAMEDICINE
Content Review
Content Self-Evaluation

Chapter 1: Introduction to Paramedicine

_____ 1. The highest level of prehospital emergency care provider and the leader of the prehospital emergency team is the
   A. Advanced EMT.
   B. paramedic.
   C. EMT.
   D. medical director.
   E. physician's assistant.

_____ 2. Although required to be licensed, registered, or credentialed, paramedics still may only function as approved by and under the direction of the system's medical director.
   A. True
   B. False

_____ 3. Today's paramedic functions in the role of
   A. 911 responder.
   B. public health advocate.
   C. injury and illness prevention advocate.
   D. public safety advocate.
   E. all of the above.

_____ 4. The paramedic must ensure that patients receive the best possible care, regardless of ability to pay, as part of his role as
   A. gatekeeper.
   B. facilitator.
   C. patient advocate.
   D. health resources link.
   E. clinician.

_____ 5. The foundation of the paramedic's education is structured within the
   A. 1998 DOT EMS curriculum.
   B. _EMS at the Crossroads_.
   C. _EMS Agenda for the Future_.
   D. National Registry of EMTs guidelines.
   E. 2009 DOT EMS education standards.

_____ 6. A skill that is infrequently used in your career as a paramedic should be practiced more during ongoing education.
   A. True
   B. False

_____ 7. Paramedics are unlikely to provide medical care in the primary care setting.
   A. True
   B. False

8. Characteristics typical of the paramedic include
    A. confident leadership.
    B. acting in the patient's best interest.
    C. excellent judgment.
    D. able to prioritize decisions.
    E. all of the above.

9. Which of the following is NOT an example of an expanded scope of practice for the paramedic?
    A. Critical care transport
    B. 911
    C. Industrial medicine
    D. Sports medicine
    E. Primary care

10. Paramedics have played an important role in the industrial setting, providing care on oil rigs, at movie sets, in factories, and in similar settings.
    A. True
    B. False

Chapter 2: EMS Systems

11. In a tiered EMS system, system members have contact with the patient in which order?
    A. Emergency physician, dispatcher, ALS provider, BLS provider
    B. Dispatcher, ALS provider, BLS provider, emergency physician
    C. Dispatcher, BLS provider, ALS provider, emergency physician
    D. Dispatcher, BLS provider, emergency physician, ALS provider
    E. None of the above

12. The concept of triage had its first use in prehospital medicine during
    A. the Napoleonic Wars.
    B. the U.S. Civil War.
    C. World War I.
    D. World War II.
    E. the Vietnam War.

13. The first federal initiative to begin today's modern EMS system was
    A. the Emergency Medical Services Act.
    B. the Robert Wood Johnson grants.
    C. the National Highway Safety Act.
    D. the Consolidated Omnibus Budget Reconciliation Act.
    E. the Health, Education, and Welfare Act.

14. Which of the following was NOT a component of the Emergency Medical Services Act of 1973?
    A. Communications
    B. Standardized recordkeeping
    C. Personnel training
    D. Medical direction
    E. System evaluation

15. The medical director is a physician who has the responsibility to be an advocate for the system to the medical community and an advocate for quality patient care.
    A. True
    B. False

16. *EMS at the Crossroads* was released in 2006 and identified key areas in which the national EMS system needs improvement.
    A. True
    B. False

17. Enhanced 911 provides which of the following?
    A. Automatic listing of the caller's location
    B. Instant routing to the appropriate agency

©2013 Pearson Education, Inc.
Paramedic Care: Principles & Practice, Vol. 1, 4th Ed.

    C. Instant call-back capability

    D. All of the above

    E. None of the above

_____ **18.** Priority dispatching is best described as

    A. using medically approved protocols to determine response configuration.

    B. giving of prearrival instructions.

    C. ensuring ambulances are staged for response.

    D. A and B.

    E. all of the above.

_____ **19.** The learning domain associated with facts or knowledge is referred to as

    A. cognitive.   **D.** didactic.

    B. psychomotor.   **E.** dexterity.

    C. affective.

_____ **20.** The process by which an agency grants recognition to an individual who has met its qualifications is

    A. licensure.   **D.** reciprocity.

    B. certification.   **E.** graduation.

    C. registration.

_____ **21.** Which of the following is an example of a national organization that tests and verifies minimum paramedic training?

    A. National Association of EMTs

    B. National Association of EMS Physicians

    C. Department of Transportation EMS Division

    D. National Registry of EMTs

    E. International Association of Flight Paramedics

_____ **22.** Through the National Registry of EMTs, individuals have access to a process tool by which they may receive reciprocity when moving from one state to another.

    A. True

    B. False

_____ **23.** What organization was established following the 9/11 terrorist attacks to help coordinate and standardize disaster response?

    A. U.S. Department of Transportation EMS Division

    B. Federal Emergency Management Association

    C. Department of Health and Human Services

    D. National Incident Management System

    E. National Registry of EMTs

_____ **24.** The agency responsible for establishing a standard list of ALS supplies and equipment for ambulances is the

    A. American College of Surgeons.

    B. American College of Emergency Physicians.

    C. Federal General Services Administration.

    D. Military Assistance to Traffic and Safety Group.

    E. National Department of Transportation.

_____ **25.** A hospital designated as a receiving facility for the EMS system should have

    A. an emergency department.

    B. 24-hour emergency physician coverage.

    C. a documented desire to participate in the system.

    D. desire to participate in multiple-casualty preparedness plans.

    E. all of the above.

_____ 26. Which of the following is NOT a part of a well-designed disaster plan?
   A. A diverse, noncentralized oversight approach
   B. Cooperation that supersedes geographical, political, and historical boundaries
   C. Frequent disaster plan tests and drills
   D. Integration of all system components
   E. All of the above

_____ 27. Which of the following is NOT one of the rules of evidence used to evaluate a proposed change in the EMS system?
   A. There must be a theoretical basis for the change.
   B. There must be scientific research to support the change.
   C. The change must be clinically important.
   D. The change must be affordable, practical, and teachable.
   E. The change must be approved by a majority of EMS practitioners.

_____ 28. In emergency medical service, customer satisfaction can be created or destroyed with a simple word or deed.
   A. True
   B. False

_____ 29. In the future, the ability of research to demonstrate the value of prehospital care may be essential to the survival of EMS.
   A. True
   B. False

_____ 30. High-risk opportunities for medical errors include
   A. skill-based failures.
   B. rules-based failures.
   C. knowledge-based failures.
   D. hand-off times.
   E. all of the above.

Chapter 3: Roles and Responsibilities of the Paramedic

_____ 31. As a paramedic, you will often serve people who are unaware of your knowledge and skills.
   A. True
   B. False

_____ 32. A paramedic unit answering which of the following calls is LEAST likely to require additional assistance?
   A. A motor vehicle collision
   B. Reported use of a weapon
   C. A single patient with a medical illness
   D. A hazardous-materials spill
   E. Rescue situations

_____ 33. Which of the following is NOT a component of the scene size-up?
   A. Identifying potential scene hazards
   B. Identifying the number of patients
   C. Applying a cervical collar
   D. Requesting additional services
   E. Determining the mechanism of injury

_____ 34. Specialty centers to which you may direct patients include which of the following?
   A. Obstetric care centers
   B. Trauma care centers
   C. Stroke care centers
   D. Burn care centers
   E. All of the above

©2013 Pearson Education, Inc.
Paramedic Care: Principles & Practice, Vol. 1, 4th Ed.

_____ 35. The highest level of trauma center is
   A. level I.   D. level IV.
   B. level II.   E. none of the above.
   C. level III.

_____ 36. Which of the following is a statement of opinion that should NOT be included on a patient-care report?
   A. "The patient was intoxicated."
   B. "The patient had the odor of alcohol on his breath."
   C. "The patient's speech was slurred."
   D. "The patient had difficulty walking."
   E. "The patient used inappropriate language when speaking."

_____ 37. As the volume of EMS responses decreases, so should the hours of training.
   A. True
   B. False

_____ 38. The paramedic who wishes to maintain interest in EMS and maintain skills and knowledge might participate in
   A. in-hospital rotations.   D. professional EMS organizations.
   B. quality improvement activities. E. all of the above.
   C. research projects.

_____ 39. In general, a profession has
   A. established standards.
   B. a specialized body of knowledge.
   C. requirements for ongoing education.
   D. requirements for initial education.
   E. all of the above.

_____ 40. The paramedic should always place the needs of the patient above his own needs.
   A. True
   B. False

Chapter 4: Workforce Safety and Wellness

_____ 41. The core elements of physical fitness are
   A. muscular strength, speed, and agility.
   B. muscular strength, good reflexes, and speed.
   C. speed, cardiovascular endurance, and flexibility.
   D. speed, cardiovascular endurance, and agility.
   E. muscular strength, cardiovascular endurance, and flexibility.

_____ 42. Active exercise performed while moving muscles through their range of motion is called
   A. isometric.   D. isotonic.
   B. polymeric.   E. anaerobic.
   C. aerobic.

_____ 43. The target heart rate is
   A. your ideal resting heart rate.
   B. your objective heart rate 5 minutes after exercise.
   C. an indicator of good cardiovascular exercise.
   D. a rate to achieve through exercise three times per week.
   E. both C and D.

_____ 44. Good nutrition is fundamental because food is your fuel.
   A. True
   B. False

_____ 45. Which of the following is NOT a major food group?
- A. Grains/bread
- B. Dairy products
- C. Carbohydrates
- D. Meat/fish
- E. None of the above

_____ 46. Which of the following is NOT recommended by the USDA as a part of diet and exercise guidelines?
- A. Chocolate and caffeine
- B. Meat and beans
- C. Fruits and vegetables
- D. Whole grains
- E. Milk

_____ 47. The old fashioned sit-up, practiced daily and in moderation, is very helpful in reducing the incidence of back injury.
- A. True
- B. False

_____ 48. Which of the following is NOT part of proper lifting?
- A. Positioning the load as close to the body as possible
- B. Keeping your feet far apart
- C. Keeping your back as straight as possible
- D. Exhaling during the lift
- E. Keeping your palms up

_____ 49. Only those patients with diagnosed HIV/AIDS, hepatitis B, and tuberculosis should be considered infectious and require you to use Standard Precautions procedures.
- A. True
- B. False

_____ 50. Which of the following items of personal protective equipment would you use with all patients?
- A. Gloves
- B. Eyewear and mask
- C. Gowns
- D. A and B
- E. A and C

_____ 51. Which of the following items of personal protective equipment are recommended when intubating a patient?
- A. Gloves
- B. Eyewear and mask
- C. Gowns
- D. A and B
- E. A, B, and C

_____ 52. HEPA and N-95 respirators are to be used when suctioning, intubating, or providing nebulized treatments or just routine care for patients who have or are suspected of having
- A. HIV/AIDS.
- B. hepatitis A.
- C. hepatitis B.
- D. tuberculosis.
- E. bacterial meningitis.

_____ 53. Gowns are recommended for which of the following situations?
- A. Intubation
- B. Splashing blood
- C. Suctioning
- D. Childbirth
- E. B and D

_____ 54. Disinfection of EMS equipment is most frequently done using
- A. bleach.
- B. radiation.
- C. chemical agents.
- D. pressurized steam.
- E. an autoclave.

_____ 55. Which of the following places the progressive stages of grieving in the correct order as you would expect to observe them in a patient?
- A. Denial, anger, bargaining, depression, acceptance
- B. Denial, bargaining, anger, depression, acceptance

C. Anger, denial, bargaining, acceptance, depression

D. Anger, denial, bargaining, depression, acceptance

E. Depression, anger, denial, bargaining, acceptance

_____ 56. A patient experiencing a major loss who puts off dealing with the event is most likely in which stage of loss?

A. Denial

B. Anger

C. Depression

D. Bargaining

E. Acceptance

_____ 57. Which age group will most likely seek out a detailed explanation of death and its difference from just being sick?

A. Newborn to age 3

B. Ages 3 to 6

C. Ages 6 to 9

D. Ages 9 to 12

E. Ages 12 to 18

_____ 58. When informing the family of the death of a member, use the words "moved on" or "has gone to a better place" rather than being blunt and using the words "dead" or "died."

A. True

B. False

_____ 59. The human response to stress progresses through three stages. They occur in which order?

A. Alarm, resistance, exhaustion

B. Resistance, alarm, exhaustion

C. Alarm, exhaustion, resistance

D. Resistance, exhaustion, alarm

E. Exhaustion, alarm, resistance

_____ 60. The condition in which coping mechanisms can no longer buffer personal job stressors is called

A. a critical incident.

B. professional overload.

C. stress.

D. disorientation.

E. burnout.

_____ 61. Which of the following is NOT a healthy behavior to help deal with or reduce stress?

A. Controlled breathing

B. Taking a few days off

C. Reframing

D. Having a few drinks to help put it behind you

E. Creating a non-EMS circle of friends

_____ 62. An example of an event that is likely to be stressful for an EMS provider is

A. suicide of an EMS worker.

B. death of a child.

C. bad incident that draws media attention.

D. serious accident with prolonged extrication.

E. all of the above.

_____ 63. Recent evidence suggests that critical stress debriefing does not appear to mitigate the effects of traumatic stress.

A. True

B. False

_____ 64. In some societies, lack of eye contact is considered a sign of respect.

A. True

B. False

_____ 65. Death and disability are common results of ambulance crashes when patients are not well secured and care providers do not wear seat belts.
A. True
B. False

Chapter 5: EMS Research

_____ 66. Originally, EMS practices and clinical procedures were based upon outcomes-based clinical research.
A. True
B. False

_____ 67. In 2001, the National EMS Research Agenda recommended that EMS
A. develop a cadre of EMS researchers.
B. establish a reliable funding stream for EMS research.
C. enhance ethical approaches to EMS research.
D. recognize the need for EMS research.
E. all of the above.

_____ 68. The first step in the scientific method is to
A. observe and ask questions.
B. determine what is already known.
C. develop a hypothesis.
D. develop a study question.
E. design an experiment.

_____ 69. Research that describes phenomena in numbers is called
A. mixed research.
B. qualitative research.
C. quantitative research.
D. variable research.
E. statistical research.

_____ 70. Prospective research begins on a specific day and lasts until a targeted end date or until a predetermined number of data points has been entered.
A. True
B. False

_____ 71. During a double-blind controlled trial, the only person who knows who is actually receiving a therapy is the
A. patient.
B. test administrator.
C. institutional review board.
D. principal investigator or statistics team.
E. none of the above.

_____ 72. A study in which various groups are compared without a control is called a
A. cohort study.
B. cross-sectional study.
C. case series.
D. _in vivo_ study.
E. _in vitro_ study.

_____ 73. What level of evidence would be assigned to the collective expert opinion of a group of recognized field experts?
A. IIa
B. IIb
C. III

©2013 Pearson Education, Inc.
Paramedic Care: Principles & Practice, Vol. 1, 4th Ed.

D. IV

E. None of the above

_____ **74.** Which of the following is a descriptive statistic?
  A. Mode
  B. Sampling error
  C. Population
  D. Confidence interval
  E. Parameters

_____ **75.** The brief paragraph that highlights the need, methods, and results of a research study is the
  A. summary.
  B. discussion.
  C. conclusion.
  D. introduction.
  E. abstract.

_____ **76.** The section of a research paper that interprets and explains the significance of research results is the
  A. summary.
  B. discussion.
  C. conclusion.
  D. introduction.
  E. abstract.

_____ **77.** What class is assigned to a treatment that is not beneficial and potentially harmful to a patient?
  A. Class I
  B. Class IIa
  C. Class IIb
  D. Class III
  E. Class X

_____ **78.** A statement claiming no difference between the results from two study groups is known as a
  A. hypothesis.
  B. prediction.
  C. theory.
  D. null hypothesis.
  E. result.

_____ **79.** The value that predicts the odds of something happening by chance alone is the
  A. p value.
  B. t value.
  C. t test.
  D. beta test.
  E. null hypothesis.

_____ **80.** Future decisions over what practices will and will not be utilized by prehospital providers will be made based upon
  A. medical director opinion.
  B. historical practices.
  C. evidence-based decisions.
  D. paramedic preferences.
  E. supply costs.

Chapter 6: Public Health

_____ **81.** Public health protects and improves community health through
  A. health education.
  B. communicable disease control.
  C. environmental hazard monitoring.
  D. preventive medicine.
  E. all of the above.

_____ **82.** Injury prevention programs that focus on keeping an injury from ever occurring are examples of
  A. primary prevention.
  B. secondary prevention.
  C. tertiary prevention.

D. acute prevention.

E. none of the above.

_____ 83. Other than the survivors and their families, no one experiences the aftermath of trauma more directly than EMS providers; hence those providers are prime candidates to be advocates of injury prevention.

A. True

B. False

_____ 84. Under the guidelines of the Occupational Safety and Health Administration (OSHA), responsibility for Standard Precautions is borne by

A. the employee.

B. the health department.

C. the state EMS authority.

D. the employer.

E. both the employer and employee.

_____ 85. Which of the following is NOT essential to safe emergency driving?

A. Being familiar with and obeying the traffic laws

B. Understanding the capabilities and limitations of the vehicle

C. Being able to drive at high speed in all conditions

D. Using proper sound and visual warning devices

E. All of the above

_____ 86. Which of the following is NOT true of premature and low-birth-weight infants?

A. There are close to 300,000 of them born each year

B. They are far more likely to die in the first year of life

C. More than 4,000 of them die each year

D. Very few have resulting disabilities

E. Their conditions often result from inadequate prenatal care

_____ 87. In children, the percentage of firearm injuries that are unintentional is about

A. 10 percent.   **D.** 30 percent.

B. 15 percent.   **E.** 33 percent.

C. 25 percent.

_____ 88. Alcohol use is a factor in about what percentage of auto collisions?

A. 10 percent

B. 20 percent

C. 25 percent

D. 40 percent

E. 50 percent

_____ 89. The early release of patients from health care facilities to help control heath care costs is NOT likely to cause an increase in the number of EMS responses.

A. True

B. False

_____ 90. An action the EMS responder can take to implement injury prevention strategies might be to

A. preserve response team safety.

B. recognize scene hazards.

C. engage in on-scene education.

D. know available community resources.

E. all of the above.

©2013 Pearson Education, Inc.
Paramedic Care: Principles & Practice, Vol. 1, 4th Ed.

Chapter 7: Medical/Legal Aspects of Prehospital Care

_____ 91. Moral responsibilities are best described as
   A. requirements of case law.
   B. requirements of statutory law.
   C. standards of a profession.
   D. personal feelings of right and wrong.
   E. legal concepts of right and wrong.

_____ 92. The term "judge-made law" is another name for
   A. constitutional law.
   B. common law.
   C. legislative law.
   D. administrative law.
   E. criminal law.

_____ 93. The regulations that permit a governmental agency to implement statutes are examples of
   A. constitutional law.
   B. common law.
   C. legislative law.
   D. administrative law.
   E. criminal law.

_____ 94. The type of law that limits the authority of the government is
   A. constitutional law.
   B. common law.
   C. legislative law.
   D. administrative law.
   E. criminal law.

_____ 95. The division of the legal system that deals with conflicts between two or more parties such as contract disputes and matrimonial issues is
   A. administrative law.
   B. criminal law.
   C. civil law.
   D. legislative law.
   E. constitutional law.

_____ 96. The individual initiating civil litigation is referred to as the
   A. victim.
   B. plaintiff.
   C. defendant.
   D. initiator.
   E. damagee.

_____ 97. Which of the following is NOT a component of a paramedic's scope of practice?
   A. Protocols
   B. System policies and procedures
   C. Certification
   D. Training and continuing education
   E. On-line medical direction

_____ 98. The degree of care, skill, and judgment that would be expected under like or similar circumstances by a similarly trained, reasonable paramedic is best defined as
   A. duty to act.
   B. standard of care.
   C. breach of duty.
   D. proximate cause.
   E. malfeasance.

_____ 99. A paramedic's action or inaction that immediately caused or worsened damages suffered by a patient is referred to as being
   A. the proximate cause.
   B. _res ipsa loquitur._
   C. a wrongful tort.
   D. actual damages.
   E. negligible.

_____ 100. If your employer or agency carries insurance coverage, you are NOT encouraged to purchase your own because your employer's or agency's coverage is most likely adequate.
   A. True
   B. False

_____ 101. Disclosing confidential patient information may expose the paramedic to litigation for
   A. defamation of character.
   B. breach of confidentiality.

C. invasion of privacy.
D. libel or slander.
E. all of the above.

____102. The act of injuring an individual's character, name, or reputation by false spoken statements with malicious intent is called
A. slander.
B. breach of confidentiality.
C. malfeasance.
D. misfeasance.
E. libel.

____103. Before beginning to treat a conscious, alert, and rational patient, you must obtain expressed consent.
A. True
B. False

____104. To give informed consent, the patient must be told and understand
A. the nature of the illness or injury.
B. the nature of the recommended treatment.
C. the risks of the recommended treatment.
D. the dangers of refusing the treatment.
E. all of the above.

____105. A patient who has once given consent may withdraw it at any time.
A. True
B. False

____106. Which of the following would NOT be considered an emancipated minor?
A. A married teenager
B. A pregnant teenager
C. A financially independent teenager living at his parent's home
D. A parent
E. A member of the armed forces

____107. Which of the following patients can refuse care?
A. A severely intoxicated patient
B. A minor
C. A conscious, alert, and rational adult
D. A patient who does not understand the intended treatment
E. A patient who does not understand the risks of treatment

____108. If you leave a patient at the emergency department without ensuring that the staff is able to continue your care, you may be guilty of
A. negligence.
B. abandonment.
C. malfeasance.
D. nonfeasance.
E. assault.

____109. The unlawful act of placing another person in fear of bodily harm is
A. assault. **D.** slander.
B. abandonment. **E.** libel.
C. battery.

____110. If you need to use force to restrain a patient, it is best to achieve it without the assistance of the police, because they are often associated with punishment.
A. True
B. False

©2013 Pearson Education, Inc.
Paramedic Care: Principles & Practice, Vol. 1, 4th Ed.

_____111. For which of the following patients would you attempt resuscitation?
  A. One who is obviously dead
  B. One with a valid DNR order
  C. One with obvious tissue decomposition
  D. One who has extreme dependent lividity
  E. None of the above

_____112. If there is any doubt about the authenticity or applicability of a DNR order, you should initiate resuscitation.
  A. True
  B. False

_____113. At the crime scene, the paramedic's primary responsibility is to protect evidence and then to treat the patient.
  A. True
  B. False

_____114. Which of the following statements regarding a paramedic's responsibility at the crime scene is NOT true?
  A. Contact law enforcement if they are not on the scene.
  B. Do not enter the crime scene unless it is safe.
  C. The paramedic's primary responsibility is patient care.
  D. Take no action to preserve evidence at the crime scene because patient care is most important.
  E. Document the movement of any scene item.

_____115. Which of the following is NOT required when documenting a patient-care response?
  A. Complete documentation promptly.
  B. Ensure it is accurate.
  C. Ensure it is objective.
  D. Maintain patient confidentiality.
  E. Ensure it is concise and brief.

Chapter 8: Ethics in Paramedicine

_____116. Which of the following might lead to ethical problems?
  A. Patients refusing care
  B. Advanced directives
  C. Hospital destinations
  D. Confidentiality
  E. All of the above

_____117. Ethics go beyond examining what is right and wrong to consider what is right or good behavior.
  A. True
  B. False

_____118. Most codes of ethics for professional groups address broad humanitarian concerns and professional etiquette.
  A. True
  B. False

_____119. When faced with an ethical challenge, which of the following is the best guiding question a paramedic can ask himself?
  A. "How would I like to be treated?"
  B. "What is in the best interest of the patient?"
  C. "Which actions will account for the greatest good?"
  D. "What would the patient want?"
  E. "What would my supervisor do?"

_____120. The term referring to the paramedic's obligation to treat all patients fairly is
A. benevolence.
B. justice.
C. beneficence.
D. autonomy.
E. euphylanthropnia.

_____121. The Latin phrase *primum non nocere* is an excellent summation of the concept of
A. beneficence.
B. autonomy.
C. justice.
D. nonmaleficence.
E. none of the above.

_____122. Which of the following is the question that best represents the interpersonal justifiability test for analyzing an ethical situation?
A. "Can you justify this action to others?"
B. "Would you want this procedure if you were in the patient's place?"
C. "Would you want this procedure performed on you if you were in similar circumstances?"
D. "Will you likely be questioned about the need for this procedure later?"
E. none of the above

_____123. When presented with a valid DNR order, the paramedic should
A. begin resuscitation immediately.
B. contact the patient's physician to verify the order's validity.
C. contact medical direction for advice before beginning resuscitation.
D. not begin resuscitation.
E. begin with CPR and delay advanced interventions.

_____124. Appropriate reasons for breaching patient confidentiality include
A. particular infectious diseases.
B. a reporter's request for information.
C. elderly neglect and abuse.
D. satisfying a coworker's curiosity.
E. A and C.

_____125. When presented with orders from a physician that do not comply with your protocols and that you believe are not in the patient's best interest, which of the following should you do?
A. Follow the physician's order and report your concerns to the medical director.
B. Ask the physician to repeat or confirm the order.
C. Ask the physician for an explanation of the order.
D. Do not follow the physician's order.
E. Do all except A.

Chapter 9: EMS System Communications

_____126. The basic communications model of exchange of information includes which of the following?
A. Sender encoding a message
B. Sender transmitting a message
C. Receiver decoding a message
D. Receiver providing feedback
E. All of the above

_____127. The radio band that penetrates buildings and is less susceptible to interference is
A. VHF low band.
B. VHF high band.
C. UHF.
D. microwave.
E. none of the above.

©2013 Pearson Education, Inc.
Paramedic Care: Principles & Practice, Vol. 1, 4th Ed.

_____128. The prehospital care report should NOT be used by
A. administration for billing.
B. the emergency department staff to identify your patient findings.
C. quality assurance committees to improve system function.
D. other paramedics to identify your interesting calls.
E. the insurance department for billing.

_____129. The phase of the emergency communications system that uses the telephone most heavily is
A. detection and citizen access.
B. the emergency response.
C. call coordination and incident recording.
D. discussion with medical direction.
E. transfer communications.

_____130. The system that uses caller questioning and established guidelines to determine the types of units that respond to a particular emergency is
A. system status management.
B. priority dispatching.
C. code identification.
D. EMD.
E. none of the above.

_____131. The radio transmission design that does NOT permit the receiver to interrupt the caller while he is talking is
A. simplex.   D. trunking.
B. duplex.   E. none of the above.
C. multiplex.

_____132. Which of the following is NOT true regarding digital communication?
A. It is clearer than analog.
B. It is faster than analog.
C. It may increase overcrowding of radio frequencies.
D. It cannot be monitored by a standard scanner.
E. It is becoming increasingly popular for EMS communications.

_____133. All of the following are appropriate for good emergency medical services communications EXCEPT
A. speaking close to the microphone.
B. speaking across or directly into the microphone.
C. talking in a loud voice.
D. speaking without emotion.
E. avoiding the use of slang or profanity.

_____134. Repeating an important order to ensure it is understood correctly is
A. redundancy.   D. reiteration.
B. multiplexing.   E. either B or D.
C. the echo procedure.

_____135. The Federal Communications Commission is responsible for all of the following EXCEPT
A. assigning and licensing radio frequencies.
B. establishing technical standards for radio equipment.
C. monitoring radio frequencies for proper use.
D. formulating acceptable medical information formats.
E. spot-checking radio base stations for proper licensing and records.

Chapter 10: Documentation

_____136. The prehospital care report should contain all of the following EXCEPT
    A. a description of your patient's condition when you arrived.
    B. a description of your patient's condition after interventions.
    C. the medical status of your patient upon arrival at the emergency department.
    D. subjective opinions about the patient's dress or actions.
    E. all of the above.

_____137. Which of the following abbreviations represents patient history?
    A. PE
    B. HH
    C. H
    D. Hx
    E. A and D

_____138. Which of the following abbreviations represents alcohol use by the patient?
    A. AOB   D. OH+
    B. ASHD   E. None of the above
    C. ETOH

_____139. Which of the following abbreviations is an indication for administering something as needed?
    A. a.c.   D. prn
    B. stat   E. WNL
    C. npo

_____140. Which of the following is NOT an example of a pertinent negative?
    A. No respiratory distress in an MI patient
    B. Nonreactive pupils in a head-injury patient
    C. Clear breath sounds in a congestive heart failure patient
    D. No history of epilepsy in seizing patient
    E. No pitting edema in a congestive heart failure patient

_____141. It is better to rephrase a patient's statement regarding history or a symptom, making it more medically correct, than to report it verbatim.
    A. True
    B. False

_____142. The best time and place to complete the prehospital report form is
    A. at the scene, if possible.
    B. in the ambulance, en route to the hospital.
    C. at the hospital before you end patient care.
    D. at the hospital after you end patient care.
    E. at the station after the call.

_____143. The best way to add information to the prehospital care report after it has been submitted to the hospital is to
    A. search and make changes on all copies.
    B. change only the original report.
    C. create an addendum and add it to all reports.
    D. not do so—never add any material to the report once submitted.
    E. make notes only on your personal copy for future reference.

_____144. The recommended way of making a correction to a prehospital care report is to
    A. draw a line through the error and initial it.
    B. erase the error completely.
    C. draw up a new form.
    D. blacken the error so it is unreadable.
    E. any of the above.

©2013 Pearson Education, Inc.
Paramedic Care: Principles & Practice, Vol. 1, 4th Ed.

_____ **145.** Which of the following is subjective patient information?
    A. Mechanism of injury
    B. Lung sounds
    C. Blood pressure
    D. Signs of injury
    E. All of the above

_____ **146.** Which of the following is objective patient information?
    A. Chief complaint
    B. Past medical history
    C. Vital signs
    D. Patient description of what happened
    E. All of the above

_____ **147.** The phrase "possible angina" in the assessment management section of a PCR is best described as
    A. the patient's presenting problem.
    B. the differential field diagnosis.
    C. the field diagnosis.
    D. a pertinent negative.
    E. both A and C.

_____ **148.** Under which element of the SOAP format would you place the patient's chief complaint?
    A. Subjective
    B. Objective
    C. Assessment
    D. Plan
    E. None of the above

_____ **149.** Under which element of the SOAP format would you place your field diagnosis?
    A. Subjective
    B. Objective
    C. Assessment
    D. Plan
    E. None of the above

_____ **150.** Under which element of the CHART format would you place standing orders?
    A. C   **D.** R
    B. H   **E.** T
    C. A

_____ **151.** The system of documentation that records information based upon time and sequence of events is the
    A. SOAP format.
    B. CHART format.
    C. patient management format.
    D. call incident approach.
    E. either B or D.

_____ **152.** When a patient refuses care against your advice, you must be sure to document that
    A. the patient is alert, oriented, and competent to make the decision.
    B. you have clearly explained the risks of not receiving care.
    C. you have tried to convince the patient to obtain care.
    D. you have explained that if the condition worsens, the patient should seek immediate care.
    E. all of the above.

_____ **153.** If you arrive at the scene of a call and are told that your services are not needed, you should
    A. simply return to service, with no need to complete a PCR.
    B. simply write "not needed" on the front of the PCR.
    C. identify any canceling authority and the time on the PCR.
    D. secure the name of the patient as well as any other information, such as the SAMPLE history.
    E. all of the above.

_____**154.** Triage tags used for a mass-casualty incident usually record

    A. vital patient information.

    B. patient priority for care and transport.

    C. all minor injuries.

    D. hospital destination.

    E. both A and B.

_____**155.** The utilization of electronic patient-care records

    A. is improving data collection.

    B. assures report legibility.

    C. provides for consistent reporting.

    D. streamlines quality assurance.

    E. all of the above.

©2013 Pearson Education, Inc.
Paramedic Care: Principles & Practice, Vol. 1, 4th Ed.

WORKBOOK ANSWER KEY

Note: Throughout Answer Key, textbook page references are shown in italic.

Chapter 1: Introduction Paramedicine

CONTENT SELF-EVALUATION

MULTIPLE CHOICE

1.	D	*p. 3*	**6.**	B	*p. 5*	**11.**	B	*p. 9*
2.	A	*p. 4*	**7.**	A	*p. 3*	**12.**	C	*p. 4*
3.	B	*p. 4*	**8.**	C	*p. 5*	**13.**	E	*p. 4*
4.	A	*p. 4*	**9.**	A	*p. 5*	**14.**	D	*p. 6*
5.	C	*p. 5*	**10.**	B	*p. 6*	**15.**	E	*p. 6*

LISTING

16. Requires an anatomy and physiology course as a prerequisite; requires a more extensive foundation of medical knowledge; provides for improved understanding of the pathophysiology of disease and injury processes. (*p. 5*)
17. **A.** advanced airway management, ventilator management, fluid and electrolyte therapy, advanced pharmacology, specialized monitoring, operating intraaortic balloon pumps, and various techniques of critical care medicine. (*p. 7*)
    B. industry-specific additional training, including knowledge and skills necessary for site safety, performing sick call duty, accident prevention, medical screening, and the administration of vaccinations and immunizations. (*p. 8*)
    C. injury care associated with the sport, injury prevention, pregame preparation, and determinations as to whether the athlete can return to practice or competition. (*p. 8*)

Chapter 2: EMS Systems

CONTENT SELF-EVALUATION

MULTIPLE CHOICE

1.	A	*p. 14*	**15.**	B	*p. 25*	**29.**	C	*p. 29*	*p. 69*
2.	A	*p. 15*	**16.**	B	*p. 26*	**30.**	B	*p. 29*	*p. 69*
3.	E	*p. 14*	**17.**	C	*p. 26*	**31.**	C	*p. 23*	*p. 72*
4.	B	*p. 14*	**18.**	A	*p. 26*	**32.**	E	*p. 31*	*p. 72*
5.	B	*p. 16*	**19.**	D	*p. 26*	**33.**	B	*p. 31*	*p. 72*
6.	B	*p. 18*	**20.**	B	*p. 27*	**34.**	C	*p. 32*	*p. 73*
7.	B	*p. 19*	**21.**	A	*p. 27*	**35.**	E	*p. 32*	*p. 73*
8.	A	*p. 23*	**22.**	D	*p. 27*	**36.**	B	*p. 32*	*p. 74*
9.	D	*p. 24*	**23.**	B	*p. 28*	**37.**	B	*p. 33*	*p. 74*
10.	C	*p. 24*	**24.**	E	*p. 28*	**38.**	A	*p. 33*	*p. 74*
11.	E	*p. 24*	**25.**	C	*p. 30*	**39.**	E	*p. 34*	*p. 76*
12.	C	*p. 24*	**26.**	B	*p. 20*	**40.**	A	*p. 35*	*p. 76*
13.	C	*p. 25*	**27.**	A	*p. 27*			
14.	A	*p. 25*	**28.**	E	*p. 22*			

LISTING

41. U.S. DOT, National Traffic and Highway Safety Administration (*p. 27*)
42. U.S. General Services Administration (*p. 29*)
43. National Registry of EMTs (*p. 28*)
44. National Academies Institute of Medicine (*p. 21*)
45. Committee on Accreditation of EMS Education Programs for the Emergency Medical Services Professional (*p. 27*)

SPECIAL PROJECT: *The EMS Agenda of the Future* (p. 20)

A. The *EMS Agenda for the Future* is a document published in 1996 creating a vision for future EMS in the United States. It identifies 14 EMS attributes and integrates EMS into the health care system.

B.
Integration of Health Services	EMS Research
Legislation and Regulation	System Finance
Human Resources	Medical Direction
Education Systems	Public Education
Prevention	Public Access
Communication Systems	Clinical Care
Information Systems	Evaluation

Chapter 3: Roles and Responsibilities of the Paramedic

CONTENT SELF-EVALUATION

MULTIPLE CHOICE

1.	A	*p. 41*	10.	B	*p. 45*	19.	B	*p. 48*
2.	E	*p. 41*	11.	C	*p. 45*	20.	B	*p. 50*
3.	E	*p. 42*	12.	C	*p. 46*	21.	A	*p. 51*
4.	A	*p. 42*	13.	E	*p. 46*	22.	D	*p. 50*
5.	E	*p. 42*	14.	E	*p. 46*	23.	A	*p. 51*
6.	D	*p. 43*	15.	B	*p. 47*	24.	E	*p. 51*
7.	E	*p. 43*	16.	B	*p. 47*	25.	C	*p. 52*
8.	B	*p. 44*	17.	B	*p. 47*			
9.	A	*p. 44*	18.	E	*p. 48*			

MATCHING

26.	J	*p. 46*	31.	A	*p. 41*	36.	G	*p. 44*
27.	F	*p. 43*	32.	D	*p. 43*	37.	A	*p. 41*
28.	G	*p. 44*	33.	E	*p. 43*	38.	J	*p. 46*
29.	C	*p. 42*	34.	H	*p. 45*	39.	C	*p. 42*
30.	I	*p. 46*	35.	B	*p. 42*	40.	E	*p. 43*

Chapter 4: Workforce Safety and Wellness

CONTENT SELF-EVALUATION

MULTIPLE CHOICE

1.	A	*p. 57*	14.	A	*p. 63*	27.	A		*p. 69*
2.	C	*p. 57*	15.	D	*p. 63*	28.	D		*p. 69*
3.	A	*p. 57*	16.	E	*p. 64*	29.	D		*p. 70*
4.	A	*p. 58*	17.	B	*p. 63*	30.	B		*p. 70*
5.	B	*p. 58*	18.	E	*p. 64*	31.	D		*p. 70*
6.	C	*p. 58*	19.	E	*p. 65*	32.	B		*p. 71*
7.	D	*p. 59*	20.	A	*p. 65*	33.	C		*p. 71*
8.	C	*p. 59*	21.	D	*p. 66*	34.	A		*p. 71, p. 69*
9.	D	*p. 60*	22.	C	*p. 67*	35.	E		*p. 71, p. 63*
10.	C	*p. 60*	23.	C	*p. 67*	36.	B		*p. 71, p. 64*
11.	A	*p. 60*	24.	B	*p. 67*	37.	E		*p. 72, p. 65*
12.	C	*p. 61*	25.	B	*p. 68*	38.	B		*p. 73, p. 65*
13.	A	*p. 62*	26.	A	*p. 68*				

MATCHING

39.	A, B	*p. 64*
40.	A, B, D	*p. 64*
41.	A, B	*p. 64*
42.	A, B, C	*p. 64*
43.	A, B, D	*p. 64*

SPECIAL PROJECT: Problem Solving pp. 66–67

1. Immediately wash the affected area with soap and water.
2. Get a medical evaluation.
3. Take the proper immunization boosters.
4. Notify the agency's infection control liaison.
5. Document the circumstances surrounding the exposure, including the actions taken to reduce chances of infection.

Chapter 5: EMS Research

CONTENT SELF-EVALUATION

MULTIPLE CHOICE

1.	E	*p. 80*	13.	C	*p. 83*	25.	D	*p. 91*
2.	B	*p. 80*	14.	A	*p. 83*	26.	A	*p. 91*
3.	D	*p. 80*	15.	B	*p. 84*	27.	D	*p. 93*
4.	A	*p. 80*	16.	B	*p. 85*	28.	C	*p. 94*
5.	E	*p. 81*	17.	A	*p. 86*	29.	C	*p. 95*
6.	D	*p. 94*	18.	B	*p. 87*	30.	A	*p. 96*
7.	A	*p. 82*	19.	D	*p. 87*	31.	E	*p. 96*
8.	B	*p. 82*	20.	E	*p. 88*			
9.	C	*p. 83*	21.	B	*p. 88*			
10.	A	*p. 83*	22.	C	*p. 88*			
11.	B	*p. 83*	23.	D	*p. 90*			
12.	E	*p. 83*	24.	E	*p. 90*			

SPECIAL PROJECT: Research Paper Critique

Answers will vary depending on article chosen.

Chapter 6: Public Health

CONTENT SELF-EVALUATION

MULTIPLE CHOICE

1.	E	*p. 101*	10.	B	*p. 106*
2.	A	*p. 100*	11.	B	*p. 107*
3.	A	*p. 102*	12.	A	*p. 107*
4.	E	*p. 100*	13.	C	*p. 101*
5.	B	*p. 102*	14.	D	*p. 103*
6.	B	*p. 103*	15.	A	*p. 107*
7.	A	*p. 103*	16.	C	*p. 107*
8.	A	*p. 105*	17.	A	*p. 108*
9.	E	*p. 106*	18.	E	*p. 108*

SPECIAL PROJECT: Research Public Health Laws

Answers will vary based on laws chosen.

Chapter 7: Medical/Legal Aspects of Prehospital Care

CONTENT SELF-EVALUATION

MULTIPLE CHOICE

1.	B	*p. 114*	13.	E	*p. 119*	25.	B	*p. 123*
2.	C	*p. 114*	14.	A	*p. 119*	26.	A	*p. 124*
3.	C	*p. 115*	15.	A	*p. 120*	27.	D	*p. 126*
4.	A	*p. 115*	16.	D	*p. 121*	28.	C	*p. 126*
5.	E	*p. 116*	17.	E	*p. 121*	29.	D	*p. 126*
6.	D	*p. 117*	18.	B	*p. 122*	30.	A	*p. 126*
7.	B	*p. 117*	19.	C	*p. 122*	31.	E	*p. 129*
8.	A	*p. 117*	20.	E	*p. 122*	32.	A	*p. 129*
9.	D	*p. 118*	21.	B	*p. 123*	33.	A	*p. 129*
10.	E	*p. 118*	22.	B	*p. 123*	34.	C	*p. 130*
11.	C	*p. 118*	23.	E	*p. 123*	35.	C	*p. 131*
12.	C	*p. 118*	24.	B	*p. 123*			

©2013 Pearson Education, Inc.
Paramedic Care: Principles & Practice, Vol. 1, 4th Ed.

¹C			²L								
O		³E	T	H	I	⁴C	S		⁵T		
M		G				I			O		
⁶M	O	R	⁷A	L		V			R		
O			⁸L	I	A	B	I	L	I	T	Y
N			B			L					
		⁹N	E	G	L	I	G	E	N	¹⁰C	E
										O	
	¹¹L	I	¹²V	I	N	G		¹³D	N	R	
¹⁴R			M							S	
I		¹⁵E	X	P	R	E	S	S	E	D	
G			L							N	
II		¹⁶T	R	I	A	L				T	
T			E								
¹⁷S	L	A	N	D	E	R					

Across

3. Rules or standards of conduct that govern members of a profession
6. Right as determined by personal conscience
8. Legal responsibility
9. Deviation from the accepted standard of care
11. _____ will: document that allows a person to specify the kinds of treatment he would desire
13. _____ order: legal document indicating the life-sustaining measures to take during cardiopulmonary arrest (abbr.)
15. _____ consent: communication from the patient indicating that he agrees to care
16. Component of a lawsuit in which both sides present testimony and evidence
17. Injuring a patient's character by false spoken statements

Down

1. _____ law: type of law derived from society's acceptance of customs and norms over time
2. Pertaining to the law
4. _____ law: division of the legal system that deals with noncriminal issues
5. A civil wrong committed by one individual against another
7. Injuring a patient's character by false written statements
10. A patient's permission to give care
12. _____ consent: type of permission to treat that is presumed from an otherwise incapacitated patient
14. Privileges that one is given by law and tradition

Chapter 8: Ethics in Paramedicine

CONTENT SELF-EVALUATION

<u>MULTIPLE CHOICE</u>

1.	A	*p. 137*	5.	D	*p. 139*	9.	A	*p. 144*
2.	B	*p. 138*	6.	B	*p. 141*	10.	E	*p. 144*
3.	D	*p. 138*	7.	A	*p. 142*			
4.	A	*p. 139*	8.	B	*p. 143*			

SPECIAL PROJECT: Ethics and the Mass-Casualty Incident

A. Although the guiding principles of health care involve doing what is in the patient's best interest (beneficence), at the mass-casualty incident the needs of multiple patients often outstrip the care resources available. Decisions must be made to ensure the most patients are benefited (justice). (*p. 144*)

B. A patient in cardiac arrest would require at least three care providers (one doing compressions, one ventilating, and one administering drugs and performing other advanced interventions). The result of an attempted resuscitation of an unwitnessed cardiac arrest patient is very likely to be poor, especially when the arrest is due to trauma. In a mass-casualty incident, the three care providers could each attend a patient (or numerous patients) who has serious injuries and increase that patient's chances for survival and reduce the seriousness of any resulting disability.

　　The triage at a mass-casualty incident presents an ethical dilemma. Prehospital care providers are taught to care for a single patient, doing all they can for him. However, at the mass-casualty incident, doing so would deny other patients the care they need. Although caring for those who would benefit most from the care does the greater good, it is hard to pass by a patient in extreme need, knowing that the lack of care ensures he will not survive. (*p. 144*)

Chapter 9: EMS System Communications

CONTENT SELF-EVALUATION

<u>MULTIPLE CHOICE</u>

1.	E	*p. 151*	12.	A	*p. 157*	23.	D	*p. 154*
2.	A	*p. 153*	13.	E	*p. 157*	24.	A	*p. 153*
3.	C	*p. 161*	14.	E	*p. 159*	25.	C	*p. 168*
4.	E	*p. 153*	15.	A	*p. 162*	26.	D	*p. 154*
5.	D	*p. 156*	16.	B	*p. 162*	27.	E	*p. 154*
6.	B	*p. 156*	17.	D	*p. 162*	28.	E	*p. 151*
7.	A	*p. 156*	18.	C	*p. 164*	29.	C	*p. 155*
8.	A	*p. 156*	19.	A	*p. 158*	30.	A	*p. 167*
9.	E	*p. 156*	20.	D	*p. 153*	31.	D	*p. 166*
10.	C	*p. 156*	21.	E	*p. 153*	32.	D	*p. 165*
11.	E	*p. 157*	22.	A	*p. 153*	33.	D	*p. 163*

Your report should include most of the following elements:

Radio message from the scene to medical direction

Unit 89 to Receiving Hospital.

We are at the ball field treating a 13-year-old male who collapsed while playing baseball. He is currently unresponsive to all but painful stimuli, is cool to the touch, and is sweating profusely. Vitals are blood pressure 136/98, pulse 92 and strong, respirations 24 and regular, and pupils equal and slow to react. ECG is showing a normal sinus rhythm. No physical signs of trauma noted, and past medical history is unknown. Oxygen is applied at 12 L via nonrebreather mask. Expected ETA, 20 minutes.

Follow-up radio message to receiving hospital

One IV in left forearm is running TKO with NS. Patient now responding to verbal stimuli. Vitals are blood pressure 134/96, pulse 90 and strong, respirations 24. ECG shows normal sinus rhythm. ETA, 10 minutes.

Ambulance run report form

Please review the accompanying form and check to be sure the form you completed includes the appropriate information. Note that you should include most, if not all, of the information listed on the accompanying sample form. If you have not done this, please review the narrative in the Workbook and determine what is missing from your version. Ensure that no important details are left out of the report.

Review the completed form on the next page to ensure that your report includes the appropriate information.

Chapter 10: Documentation

CONTENT SELF-EVALUATION

MULTIPLE CHOICE

1.	E	*p. 173*	**9.**	C	*p. 182*	**17.**	A	*p. 185*
2.	B	*p. 173*	**10.**	B	*p. 182*	**18.**	E	*p. 185*
3.	A	*p. 173*	**11.**	B	*p. 184*	**19.**	E	*p. 189*
4.	B	*p. 182*	**12.**	A	*p. 174*	**20.**	C	*p. 191*
5.	B	*p. 174*	**13.**	E	*p. 184*			
6.	E	*p. 176*	**14.**	A	*p. 184*			
7.	A	*p. 176*	**15.**	D	*p. 185*			
8.	D	*p. 176*	**16.**	E	*p. 186*			

Radio message from the scene to medical direction

Unit 21 to Medical Direction. We are attending a male victim of a one-car crash. He was initially unconscious but is now conscious, alert, and oriented. He has a small contusion on his forehead, the windshield is broken, and there is a small welt on his neck. He was stung by a bee and has had a previous allergic reaction. Vitals are blood pressure 110/76, pulse 90 and strong, respirations 30, and O_2 saturation 94 percent. There are audible wheezes, and he is complaining of "a lump in the throat." He is on 12 L of O_2 via nonrebreather mask and has one IV of LR running TKO. A cervical collar has been applied and spinal immobilization is underway.

Follow-up radio message to community hospital

0.3 mg epinephrine subcutaneously and 50 mg Benadryl IM have been administered. Current vitals are blood pressure 122/78, pulse 68 and strong, respirations 22 and regular, O_2 saturation 98 percent. Breath sounds are now clear. ETA is 10 minutes. Completed run report for Chapter 5 (page 113).

Ambulance run report form

Please check to be sure the form you completed includes the appropriate information. Please review the narrative in the Workbook and determine what may be missing from your version. Ensure that no important details are left out of the report.

Date **Today's Date**	Emergency Medical Services Run Report	Run # **911**

Patient Information / Service Information / Times

Patient Information		Service Information	Times
Name: **Thompson, Jim**		Agency: **Unit 89**	Rcvd **15:15**
Address: **Unknown**		Location: **Ball field**	Enrt **15:16**
City:	St: Zip:	Call Origin: **Dispatch**	Scne **15:22**
Age: **13** Birth: / / Sex: [**M**][F]		Type: Emrg[**X**] Non[ ] Trnsfr[ ]	LvSn **15:38**
Nature of Call: **Unconscious person**			ArHsp **15:57**
Chief Complaint: **Unconsciousness—possible heat exhaustion**			InSv **16:15**

Description of Current Problem:

The patient collapsed while playing baseball on a very hot, sunny

day. Pt. was found to be cool & diaphoretic, unresponsive to

verbal stimuli, and responsive to painful stimuli. Pupils were

normal in size but slow to react. Physical assessment reveals no

apparent signs of trauma or other medical problem.

Medical Problems

Past		Present
[ ]	Cardiac	[ ]
[ ]	Stroke	[ ]
[ ]	Acute Abdomen	[ ]
[ ]	Diabetes	[ ]
[ ]	Psychiatric	[ ]
[ ]	Epilepsy	[ ]
[ ]	Drug/Alcohol	[ ]
[ ]	Poisoning	[ ]
[ ]	Allergy/Asthma	[ ]
[ ]	Syncope	[ ]
[ ]	Obstetrical	[ ]
[ ]	GYN	[ ]

Other: **Unknown**

Trauma Scr: **n/a**   Glasgow: **6**

On-Scene Care: **provided oxygen, removed patient from sun and heat. Attempted IV in right forearm (unsuccessful) started IV in left forearm w/16 ga NS – TKO**	First Aid: **pillow was placed under head (removed by EMS)**
	By Whom? **bystanders**

O₂ @ **12** L **15:27** Via **NRB**	C-Collar **n/a** :	S-Immob. **n/a**	Stretcher **15:37**

Allergies/Meds: **Unknown**	Past Med Hx: **Unknown**

Time	Pulse	Resp.	BP S/D	LOC	ECG
15:27	R: **92** [**X**][i]	R: **24** [s][l]	**136/98**	[a][v][**X**][u]	**Normal Sinus Rhythm**
Care/Comments: **Pt. unresponsive to all but painful stimuli**					
15:37	R: **90** [**X**][i]	R: **24** [s][l]	**134/96**	[a][**X**][p][u]	**Normal Sinus Rhythm**
Care/Comments: **Pt. became responsive to verbal stimuli**					
15:45	R: **88** [**X**][i]	R: **24** [s][l]	**132/90**	[**X**][v][p][u]	**Normal Sinus Rhythm**
Care/Comments: **Pt. became fully conscious, alert, and oriented**					
:	R: [r][i]	R: [s][l]	/	[a][v][p][u]	
Care/Comments:					

Destination: **Receiving Hospital**	Personnel:	Certification
Reason: [ ]pt [**X**]Closest [ ]M.D. [ ]Other	1. **Your Name**	[**X**][E][O]
Contacted: [**X**]Radio [ ]Tele [ ]Direct	2. **Steve Phillips**	[P][**X**][O]
Ar Status: [**X**]Better [ ]UnC [ ]Worse	3. **n/a**	[P][E][O]

Introduction to Advanced Prehospital Care: Content Review

CONTENT SELF-EVALUATION

CHAPTER 1: INTRODUCTION TO PARAMEDICINE

1.	B	*p. 3*	5.	E	*p. 6*	9.	B	*p. 9*
2.	A	*p. 4*	6.	A	*p. 5*	10.	A	*p. 9*
3.	E	*p. 4*	7.	B	*p. 7*			
4.	C	*p. 4*	8.	E	*p. 5*			

CHAPTER 2: EMS SYSTEMS

11.	C	*p. 14*	18.	D	*p. 26*	25.	E	*p. 30*
12.	A	*p. 15*	19.	A	*p. 27*	26.	A	*p. 32*
13.	C	*p. 18*	20.	B	*p. 27*	27.	E	*p. 31*
14.	D	*p. 18*	21.	D	*p. 28*	28.	A	*p. 33*
15.	A	*p. 23*	22.	A	*p. 28*	29.	A	*p. 34*
16.	A	*p. 21*	23.	D	*p. 20*	30.	E	*p. 33*
17.	D	*p. 25*	24.	B	*p. 29*			

CHAPTER 3: ROLES AND RESPONSIBILITIES OF THE PARAMEDIC

31.	A	*p. 41*	35.	A	*p. 44*	39.	E	*p. 48*
32.	C	*p. 42*	36.	A	*p. 46*	40.	B	*p. 48*
33.	C	*p. 42*	37.	B	*p. 47*			
34.	E	*p. 44*	38.	E	*p. 48*			

CHAPTER 4: WORKFORCE SAFETY AND WELLNESS

41.	E	*p. 57*	50.	A	*p. 62*	59.	A	*p. 69*
42.	D	*p. 58*	51.	D	*p. 63*	60.	E	*p. 71*
43.	E	*p. 58*	52.	D	*p. 63*	61.	D	*p. 71*
44.	A	*p. 58*	53.	E	*p. 63*	62.	E	*p. 72*
45.	C	*p. 58*	54.	A	*p. 65*	63.	A	*p. 73*
46.	A	*p. 59*	55.	A	*p. 67*	64.	A	*p. 73*
47.	B	*p. 60*	56.	A	*p. 67*	65.	A	*p. 74*
48.	B	*p. 61*	57.	C	*p. 68*			
49.	B	*p. 62*	58.	B	*p. 68*			

CHAPTER 5: EMS RESEARCH

66.	B	*p. 80*	71.	D	*p. 84*	76.	B	*p. 90*
67.	D	*p. 80*	72.	B	*p. 85*	77.	D	*p. 96*
68.	A	*p. 81*	73.	D	*p. 87*	78.	D	*p. 95*
69.	C	*p. 83*	74.	A	*p. 88*	79.	A	*p. 94*
70.	A	*p. 83*	75.	E	*p. 90*	80.	C	*p. 96*

CHAPTER 6: PUBLIC HEALTH

81.	D	*p. 100*	85.	C	*p. 106*	89.	B	*p. 108*
82.	A	*p. 102*	86.	D	*p. 107*	90.	E	*p. 108*
83.	A	*p. 103*	87.	B	*p. 107*			
84.	E	*p. 105*	88.	E	*p. 107*			

CHAPTER 7: MEDICAL/LEGAL ASPECTS OF PREHOSPITAL CARE

91.	D	*p. 115*	100.	B	*p. 119*	109.	A	*p. 126*
92.	B	*p. 115*	101.	E	*p. 121*	110.	B	*p. 126*
93.	D	*p. 115*	102.	A	*p. 122*	111.	E	*p. 127*
94.	A	*p. 115*	103.	A	*p. 122*	112.	A	*p. 127*
95.	C	*p. 115*	104.	E	*p. 122*	113.	B	*p. 130*
96.	B	*p. 115*	105.	A	*p. 122*	114.	D	*p. 130*
97.	E	*p. 116*	106.	C	*p. 123*	115.	E	*p. 131*
98.	B	*p. 118*	107.	C	*p. 123*			
99.	A	*p. 119*	108.	B	*p. 126*			

CHAPTER 8: ETHICS IN PARAMEDICINE

116.	E	*p. 136*	120.	B	*p. 139*	124.	E	*p. 143*
117.	A	*p. 137*	121.	D	*p. 139*	125.	E	*p. 145*
118.	A	*p. 138*	122.	A	*p. 141*			
119.	B	*p. 138*	123.	D	*p. 141*			

CHAPTER 9: EMS SYSTEM COMMUNICATIONS

126.	E	*p. 152*	130.	B	*p. 157*	134.	C	*p. 154*
127.	C	*p. 161*	131.	A	*p. 162*	135.	D	*p. 168*
128.	D	*p. 154*	132.	C	*p. 163*			
129.	A	*p. 155*	133.	C	*p. 153*			

CHAPTER 10: DOCUMENTATION

136.	D	*p. 172*	143.	C	*p. 184*	150.	D	*p. 187*
137.	D	*p. 177*	144.	A	*p. 184*	151.	D	*p. 188*
138.	C	*p. 178*	145.	A	*p. 185*	152.	E	*p. 188*
139.	D	*p. 180*	146.	C	*p. 185*	153.	C	*p. 189*
140.	C	*p. 176*	147.	C	*p. 186*	154.	E	*p. 190*
141.	B	*p. 182*	148.	A	*p. 187*	155.	E	*p. 191*
142.	D	*p. 184*	149.	C	*p. 187*			

©2013 Pearson Education, Inc.
Paramedic Care: Principles & Practice, Vol. 1, 4th Ed.